How to Quickly and Accurately Master ECG Interpretation

DALE DAVIS, RCT
General Partner, Cardiac Educational Resources
Mendham, New Jersey

Illustrated by Patrick Turner

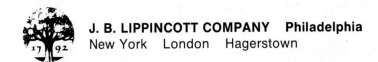

J. B. LIPPINCOTT COMPANY   Philadelphia
New York   London   Hagerstown

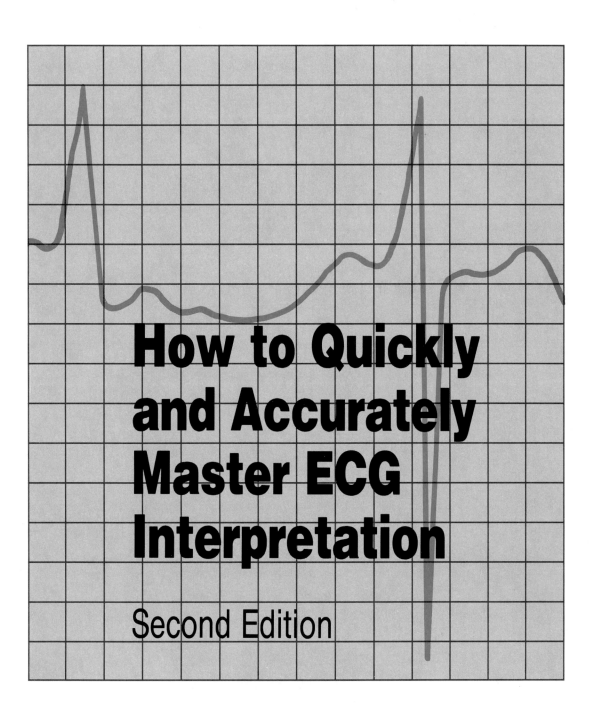

How to Quickly and Accurately Master ECG Interpretation

Second Edition

Acquisitions Editor: Charles McCormick
Sponsoring Editor: Kimberley Cox
Project Editor: Dina Kamilatos
Indexer: Victoria Boyle
Designer: Patrick Turner
Design Coordinator: Kathy Kelley-Luedtke
Production Manager: Caren Erlichman
Production Coordinator: Kathryn Rule
Compositor: Bi-Comp, Incorporated
Printer/Binder: R. R. Donnelley & Sons Company

2nd Edition

   3   5   6   4

Davis, Dale.
   How to quickly and accurately master ECG interpretation / Dale
Davis ; illustrated by Patrick Turner. — 2nd ed.
     p. cm.
   Includes bibliographical references and index.
   ISBN 0-397-51106-X
   1. Electrocardiography. 2. Heart—Diseases—Diagnosis.
I. Title.
   RC683.5.E5D33 1992
   616.1'207547—dc20

                                                  90-29999
                                                     CIP

PREFACE

How to Quickly and Accurately Master ECG Interpretation is designed as an easy yet comprehensive approach to basic ECG interpretation. What has been available to the student in the past was either a book that was much too elementary with no reference value, or a complicated ECG manual that was difficult to complete without extra help. This book is a mixture of both methods, combined into one easy-to-understand program that can be used not only for quick and comprehensive learning, but also as a reference and a study guide.

Chapters 1 through 9 cover the fundamental knowledge necessary to evaluate normal 12-lead ECGs; Chapters 10 through 13 cover the specialized criteria necessary to interpret abnormal 12-lead ECGs; and Chapters 14 and 15 allow the student to practice and sharpen the newly acquired arrhythmia interpretation skills.

The book is presented in a simply organized step-by-step learning process, and includes easy-to-understand diagrams that enhance the text and assure comprehension of the electrophysiology of the normal and abnormal ECG, rather than just memorization of criteria. I have intentionally chosen simplicity in favor of exactness in some areas of the book in order to make learning uncomplicated.

A summary of each ECG abnormality discussed in a particular chapter is presented on a two-page display at the end of the chapter and is divided into three parts:

1. A diagram of the heart demonstrates the ECG abnormality, with the ECG leads necessary for examination placed around the heart in their correct positions.
2. Criteria necessary for recognition of the abnormality are listed directly below the heart diagram.
3. A 12-lead ECG that is representative of the ECG abnormality is displayed on the opposite page, with the previously designated leads observed around the heart diagram and in the criteria section tinted in blue for final correlation.

Practice ECGs with answers comprised of interpretations that relate only to the topic discussed in the chapter are included at the end of each ECG abnormality chapter. These ECGs are designed to reinforce the one concept just learned, without the student having to concern himself with other abnormalities.

For the second edition, the 12-lead ECG examples throughout the text and at the end of each chapter have been replaced and now include the entire ECG record rather than just one representative complex from each lead. This will allow the reader to calculate the heart rate on all the ECGs and to become accustomed to interpreting an entire ECG rather than just one perfect ECG complex.

Chapter 14 has been devoted to differential diagnosis and presents an easy and organized step-by-step method for interpretation of ECGs. The criteria for the ECG abnormalities are individually examined and compared to one another to demonstrate possible identification problems and to give suggestions and hints for easier solutions. The most common interpretation pitfalls are discussed and demonstrated with 66 new 12-lead ECGs.

The intention and scope of this edition are unchanged and simplicity and an organized interpretative method still remain the central themes. I am most appreciative for the positive response to this book, and I hope that changes and additions to this edition will make learning much easier and more effective.

Dale Davis, RCT

CONTENTS

CONTENTS

How to Quickly and Accurately Master ECG Interpretation

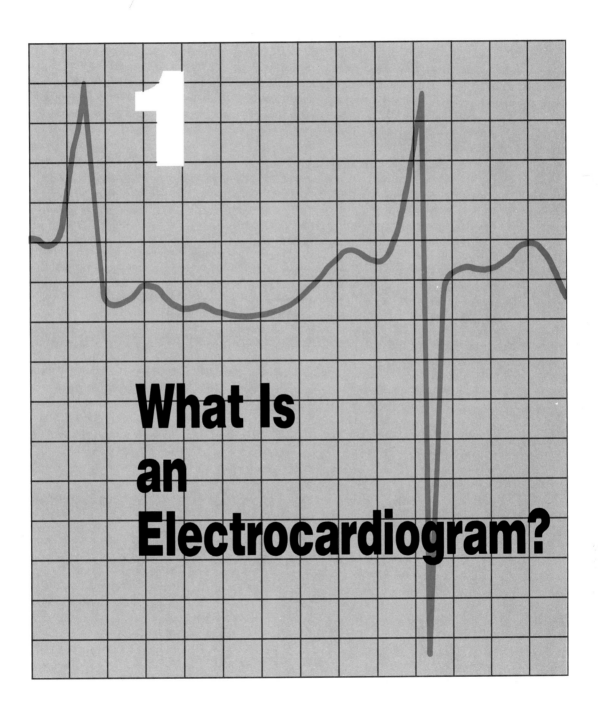

1

What Is
an
Electrocardiogram?

An electrocardiogram (ECG) is a recording of the electrical activity occurring in the heart each time it contracts.

Electrodes are placed on designated areas of the patient's body, and by the use of various combinations of these electrodes, 12 different views of the same electrical activity are demonstrated on the ECG graph paper. Each separate view of the heart is called an *ECG lead*. In routine testing we use a 12-lead ECG, consisting of three standard leads and three augmented leads that view the heart in the frontal plane, and six precordial or chest leads that view the heart in the horizontal plane.

Electrodes are placed on both the wrists and on the left ankle of the patient to obtain the standard and augmented leads, but the electrodes actually may be placed anywhere on the respective limbs or upper and lower torso, and the same view of the heart is recorded. A fourth electrode is placed on the right ankle to stabilize the ECG, but this electrode takes no part in lead formation.

STANDARD AND AUGMENTED
LEAD PLACEMENT

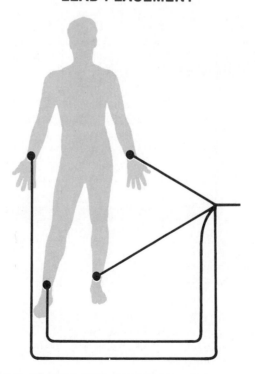

HOW TO QUICKLY AND ACCURATELY MASTER ECG INTERPRETATION

STANDARD LEADS

The standard leads are called *bipolar leads* because they are composed of two electrodes—one that is negative and one that is positive—and the ECG records the difference in electrical potential between them.

LEAD I

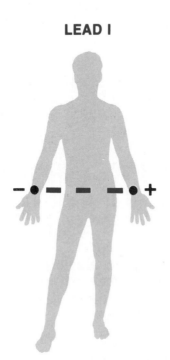

Lead I is composed of the right arm, which is designated as negative, and the left arm, which is considered positive.

LEAD II

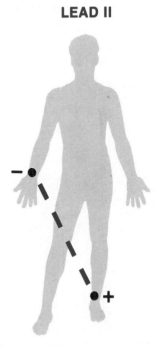

Lead II is composed of the right arm, which is made negative, and the left leg, which is considered positive.

WHAT IS AN ELECTROCARDIOGRAM?

Lead III is made up of the left arm, which is designated as negative, and the left leg, which is considered positive.

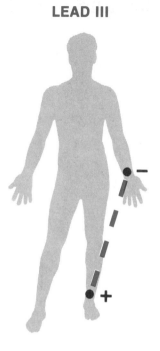

The three standard leads form a triangle over the body and have a mathematical relationship to one another as described by Einthoven: The height or depth of the recordings in lead I plus lead III equals the height or depth of the recordings in lead II.

EINTHOVEN'S TRIANGLE

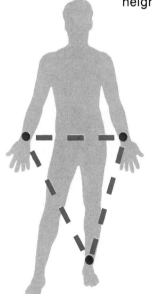

II   =   I   +   III

HOW TO QUICKLY AND ACCURATELY MASTER ECG INTERPRETATION

AUGMENTED LEADS

The same three electrodes used in the standard leads—left arm, right arm, and left leg—are used for augmented lead composition, only in different combinations. The augmented leads are considered unipolar leads because they comprise one positive electrode—either the left arm, right arm, or left leg—recording the electrical potential at that one point with reference to the other two remaining leads. Because of the manner in which these leads are arranged, the voltage is extremely low and must be augmented to equal the voltage of the remainder of the ECG. This increase is accomplished by the ECG machine.

LEAD AVR

aVR—Augmented Voltage of the Right Arm
The right arm is the positive electrode in reference to the left arm and left leg. This lead records the electrical activity of the heart from the direction of the right arm.

LEAD AVL

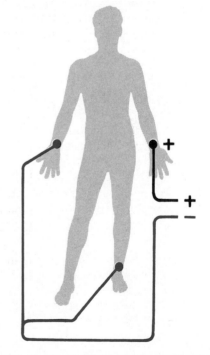

aVL—Augmented Voltage of the Left Arm
The left arm is the positive electrode in reference to the right arm and the left leg. This lead views the electrical activity of the heart from the direction of the left arm.

WHAT IS AN ELECTROCARDIOGRAM?

aVF—Augmented Voltage of the Left Foot

The left foot or the left leg is the positive electrode in reference to the left arm and the right arm. This lead sees the electrical activity of the heart from the direction of the bottom of the heart.

LEAD AVF

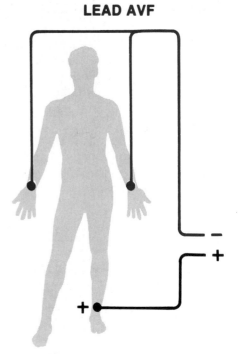

PRECORDIAL LEADS

The six precordial leads are unipolar leads and view the electrical activity of the heart in the horizontal plane. The following positions are used for placement of a suction cup lead on the chest to obtain the correct precordial lead placement:

PRECORDIAL LEAD PLACEMENT

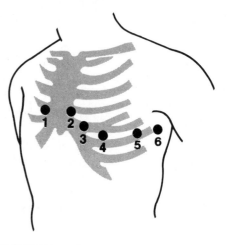

V_1 4th intercostal (between the ribs) space immediately to the right of the sternum

V_2 4th intercostal space immediately to the left of the sternum

V_3 Directly between V_2 and V_4

V_4 5th intercostal space—left midclavicular (midcollarbone) line

V_5 5th intercostal space—left anterior axillary (armpit) line

V_6 5th intercostal space—left midaxillary line

HOW TO QUICKLY AND ACCURATELY MASTER ECG INTERPRETATION

The precordial leads view the heart in the horizontal plane. Imagine sawing the body into two parts at the level of the heart and lifting off the top part of the body and looking down at the heart.

PRECORDIAL LEADS VIEW THE HEART IN THE HORIZONTAL PLANE

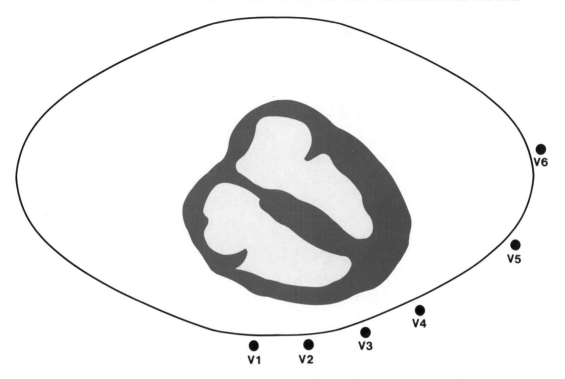

V_1 and V_2 are placed over the right ventricle.
V_3 and V_4 lie over the interventricular septum.
V_5 and V_6 are placed over the left ventricle.

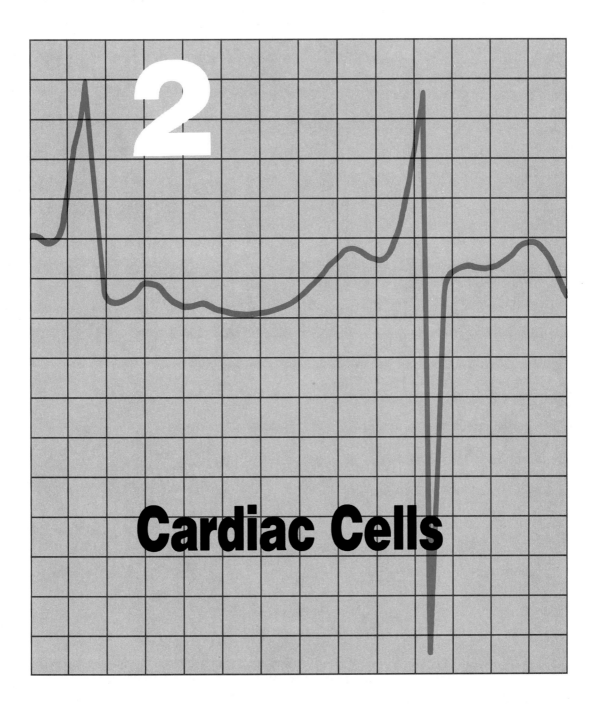

2

Cardiac Cells

DEPOLARIZATION AND REPOLARIZATION

Each cardiac cell is surrounded by and filled with a solution that contains ions. The three ions that we will be concerned with are sodium (Na^+), potassium (K^+), and calcium (Ca^{++}). In the resting period of the cell, the inside of the cell membrane is considered negatively charged, and the outside of the cell membrane is positively charged. The movement of these ions inside and across the cell membrane constitutes a flow of electricity that generates the signals on an ECG.

When an electrical impulse is initiated in the heart, the inside of a cardiac cell rapidly becomes positive in relation to the outside of the cell. The electrical impulse causing this excited state and this change of polarity is called *depolarization*. An electrical impulse begins at one end of a cardiac cell, and this wave of depolarization propagates through the cell to the opposite end. The return of the stimulated cardiac cell to its resting state is called *repolarization*. This phase of recovery allows the inside of the cell membrane to return to its normal negativity. Repolarization begins at the end of the cell that was just depolarized. The resting state is maintained until the arrival of the next wave of depolarization.

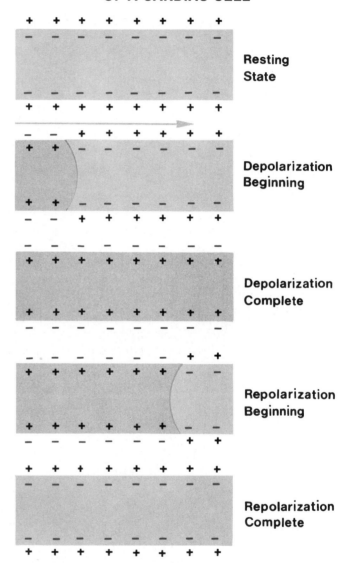

DEPOLARIZATION AND REPOLARIZATION OF A CARDIAC CELL

Resting State

Depolarization Beginning

Depolarization Complete

Repolarization Beginning

Repolarization Complete

Once the cardiac cells have been depolarized, a second wave of depolarization cannot occur until the first depolarization is completely finished. This is called the *absolute refractory period*. Immediately following this, the *relative refractory period* occurs during repolarization, at which time the cardiac cell is capable of being depolarized again but only by a strong stimulus.

ELECTROPHYSIOLOGIC PROPERTIES OF A CARDIAC CELL

Automaticity. The heart can begin and maintain rhythmic activity without the aid of the nervous system. A heart removed from the body has the ability to beat on its own for a period of time. The highest degree of automaticity is found in the pacemaker cells of the sinus node. The atria, atrioventricular (AV) node, bundle of His, bundle branches, Purkinje fibers, and the ventricular myocardium have a lesser degree of automaticity.

Excitability. A cardiac cell will respond to an electrical stimulus with an abrupt change in its electrical potential. Each cardiac cell that receives an electrical impulse will change its ionic composition and its respective polarity. Once an electrical potential begins in a cardiac cell it will continue until the entire cell is polarized.

Conductivity. A cardiac cell transfers an impulse to a neighboring cell very rapidly, so that all areas of the heart appear to depolarize at once. This principle is the same as that which applies to the electrical wiring on Christmas tree lights: The electrical wire propagates the electrical impulse to each light in succession in such a short span of time that all of the lights appear to light together. The velocity of transfer varies in the different cardiac tissues:

   200 mm per second in the AV node
   400 mm per second in ventricular muscle
   1000 mm per second in atrial muscle
   4000 mm per second in the Purkinje fibers

VELOCITY OF CONDUCTION OF ELECTRICAL IMPULSES

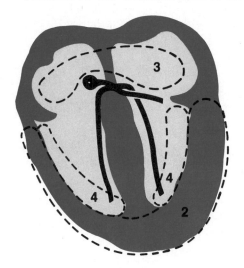

1. 200 mm/second
2. 400 mm/second
3. 1000 mm/second
4. 4000 mm/second

CARDIAC CELLS

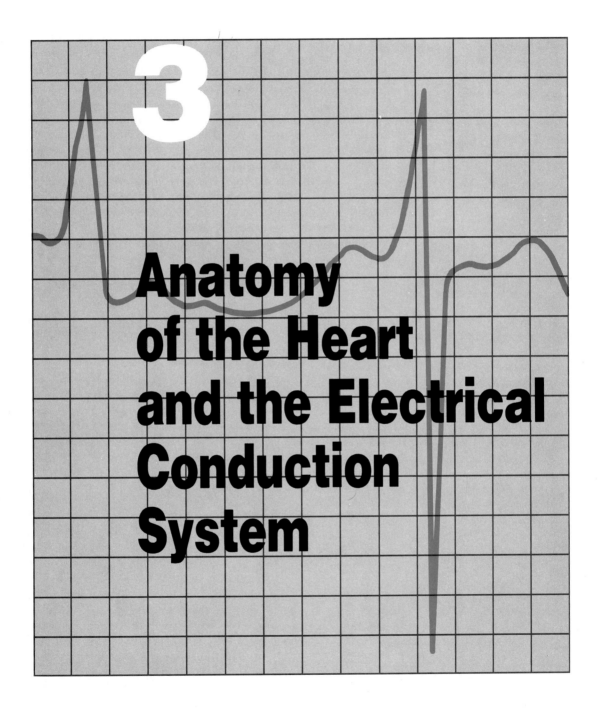

3

Anatomy of the Heart and the Electrical Conduction System

ANATOMY

The heart is a muscular organ whose ultimate purpose is to pump blood to all the tissues of the body and thus to nourish them with oxygen. This is accomplished with a four-compartment heart. The two smaller upper chambers are the receiving chambers, called the *left atrium* and *right atrium,* and are divided by a wall called the *interatrial septum*. The two lower chambers, called the *ventricles,* are divided by a thicker wall, called the *interventricular septum*. The ventricles are responsible for pumping blood out of the heart. The right ventricle pumps unoxygenated blood a very short distance to the lungs, and the left ventricle has the more demanding job of pumping oxygenated blood throughout the entire circulatory system. Therefore, the left ventricular walls must be thicker than those of the right. The walls of the heart are composed of three distinct layers: (1) the *endocardium,* which is the thin membrane lining the inside of the cardiac muscle; (2) the cardiac muscle, called the *myocardium;* and (3) the *epicardium,* which is a thin membrane lining the outside of the myocardium.

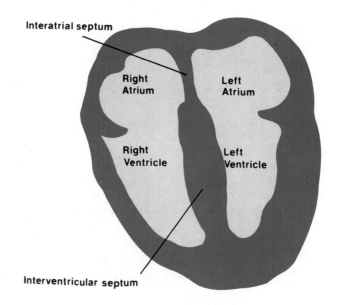

Interatrial septum

Right Atrium

Left Atrium

Right Ventricle

Left Ventricle

Interventricular septum

Unoxygenated blood is returned from the body to the right atrium. It flows into the right ventricle, where it is pumped a short distance into the lungs by way of the pulmonary artery to become oxygenated, and then is ready to be delivered back to the body. It begins its journey back by first entering the left atrium by way of the pulmonary veins. It then flows into the left ventricle and is pumped out to the entire body through the aorta to nourish the tissues with oxygen.

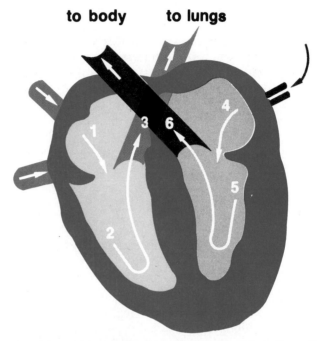

1. **Unoxygenated blood returns to the right atrium from the superior and inferior vena cava.**
2. **Blood proceeds to the right ventricle.**
3. **Blood is pumped into the pulmonary artery and into the lungs.**
4. **Oxygenated blood returns to the left atrium through pulmonary veins.**
5. **Blood flows to left ventricle.**
6. **Blood is pumped into the aorta and out to the body.**

ANATOMY OF THE HEART AND THE ELECTRICAL CONDUCTION SYSTEM

Some terms referring to anatomic position should be understood to proceed with our description of the heart:

Anterior	Toward the front
Posterior	Toward the back
Inferior	Lower
Superior	Higher
Lateral	Toward the side
Apex	The pointed end of the ventricles

If we view the heart as it is seen lying within the chest, the right atrium and ventricle are in front of or lying anterior to the left atrium and ventricle. The left atrium and ventricle are in back of or lying posterior to the right atrium and ventricle. The atria are superior to the ventricles, and the ventricles are inferior to the atria.

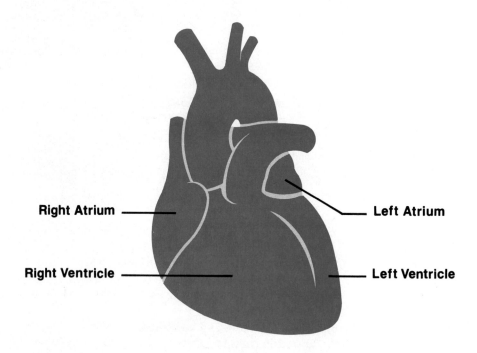

Right Atrium ——————   —————— **Left Atrium**

Right Ventricle ——————   —————— **Left Ventricle**

If we examine just the left ventricle as if we had removed it from the rest of the heart, we label the different walls of the chamber as anterior, posterior, inferior, and lateral.

ANATOMICAL AREAS OF LEFT VENTRICLE

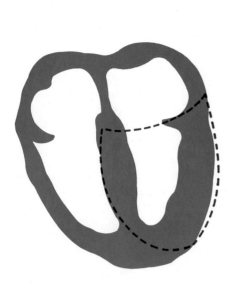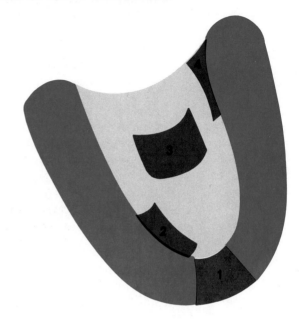

1. Anterior
2. Inferior
3. Posterior
4. Lateral

ANATOMY OF THE HEART AND THE ELECTRICAL CONDUCTION SYSTEM

ELECTRICAL CONDUCTION SYSTEM

Now that you are familiar with the heart's function of pumping blood throughout the body, you should understand what actually initiates this mechanical action.

The electrical conduction system contains all the wiring and parts necessary to initiate and maintain rhythmic contraction of the heart. The system consists of (1) the sinoatrial (SA) node, (2) the internodal pathways, (3) the AV node, (4) the bundle of His, (5) the right bundle branch and the left bundle branch and its anterior and posterior divisions, and (6) the Purkinje fibers.

SA Node. The cardiac impulse originates in the SA node, called "the pacemaker of the heart," located in the upper wall of the right atrium. The SA node has an elongated, oval shape and varies in size but is larger than the AV node.

SA NODE

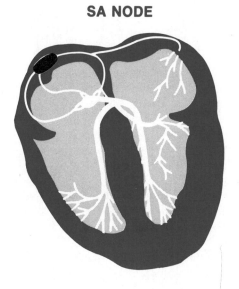

Internodal Pathways. The cardiac impulse spreads through both atria by way of the internodal pathways and causes both atria to depolarize and then to contract.

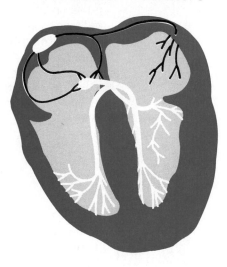

INTERNODAL PATHWAYS

AV Node. The depolarization wave arrives at the AV node, which is an oval structure approximately one third to one half the size of the SA node, and located on the right side of the interatrial septum; the wave is delayed there for approximately .10 second before arriving at the bundle of His.

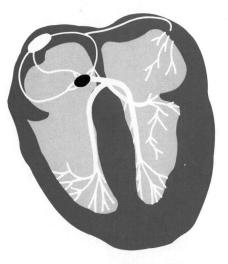

AV NODE

Bundle of His. The cardiac impulse spreads to the thin bundle of threads connecting the AV node to the bundle branches, which are located in the right side of the interatrial septum just above the ventricles.

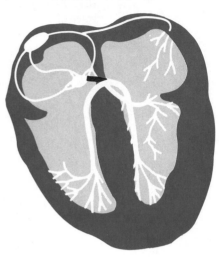

BUNDLE OF HIS

Right and Left Bundle Branches. The right bundle branch is a slender fascicle that runs along the right side of the interventricular septum and supplies the electrical impulses to the right ventricle.

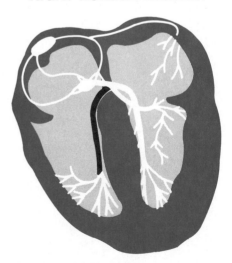

RIGHT BUNDLE BRANCH

The left bundle branch is the other branch of the bundle of His and supplies electrical impulses to the left ventricle. It runs along the left side of the interventricular septum and divides almost immediately into an anterior and a posterior division.

The Anterior Fascicle supplies the anterior and superior portions of the left ventricle with electrical impulses.

LEFT ANTERIOR FASCICLE

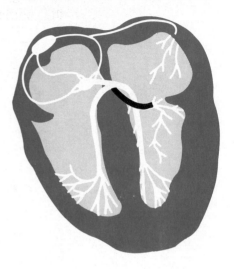

The Posterior Fascicle supplies the posterior and inferior portions of the left ventricle with electrical impulses.

LEFT POSTERIOR FASCICLE

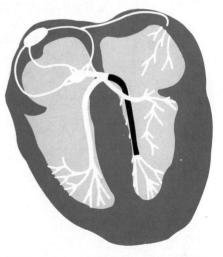

ANATOMY OF THE HEART AND THE ELECTRICAL CONDUCTION SYSTEM

Purkinje Fibers. The bundle branches both terminate in a network of fibers that are located in both the left and right ventricular walls. The cardiac impulse travels into the Purkinje fibers and causes ventricular depolarization and then ventricular contraction.

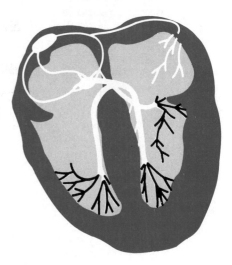

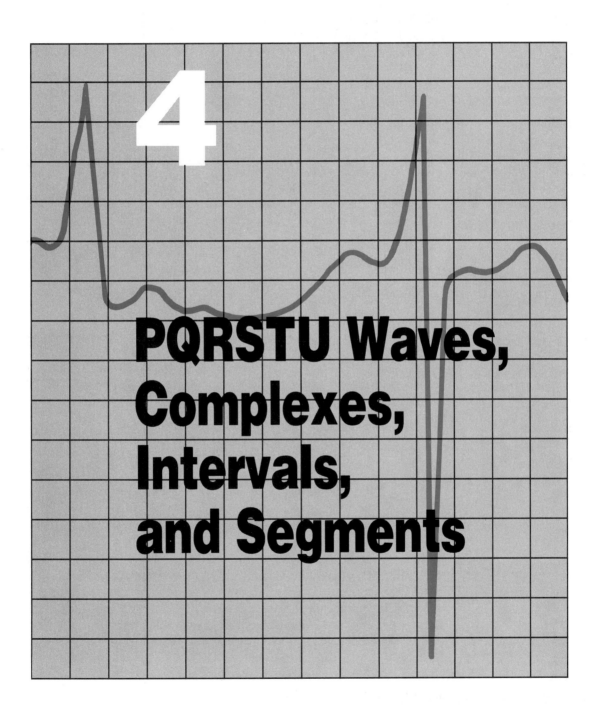

4

PQRSTU Waves, Complexes, Intervals, and Segments

The purpose of this chapter is to correlate the electrical events in the heart with the characteristic markings and configurations that occur during an ECG tracing.

WAVES AND COMPLEXES

A wave of depolarization begins in the SA node and spreads to both atria by way of the internodal pathways, and both atria depolarize. Atrial depolarization is represented by the P wave. P waves are usually upright and slightly rounded.

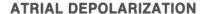

ATRIAL DEPOLARIZATION

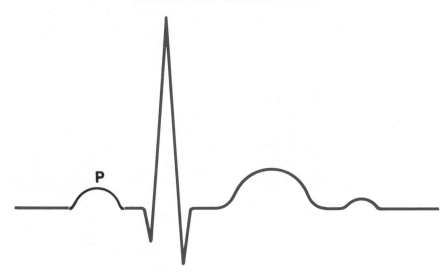

Remember, when cardiac cells depolarize they must also repolarize to regain their proper resting charge. Atrial repolarization is represented by the Ta wave, and its direction is opposite to that of the P wave. This wave is often not visible on the ECG because it usually coincides with the QRS complex and is impossible to recognize.

ATRIAL REPOLARIZATION

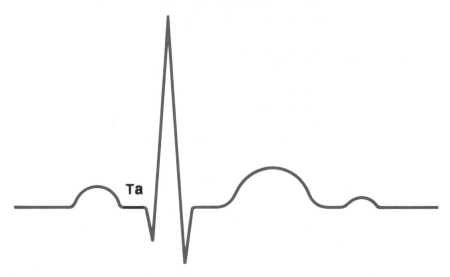

The wave of depolarization then spreads to the AV node, the bundle of His, the bundle branches, the Purkinje fibers, and the ventricular myocardium. Ventricular depolarization occurs and is represented by the QRS complex.

VENTRICULAR DEPOLARIZATION

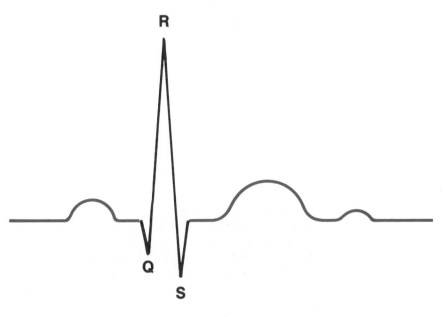

PQRSTU WAVES, COMPLEXES, INTERVALS, AND SEGMENTS

Ventricular repolarization is represented by the T wave. The T wave is normally upright and slightly rounded.

VENTRICULAR REPOLARIZATION

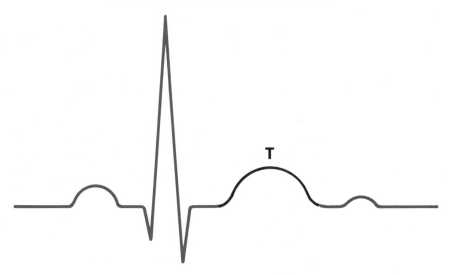

A U wave is sometimes seen after the T wave. It is thought to relate to the events of late repolarization of the ventricles. The U wave should be of the same direction as the T wave.

LATE REPOLARIZATION

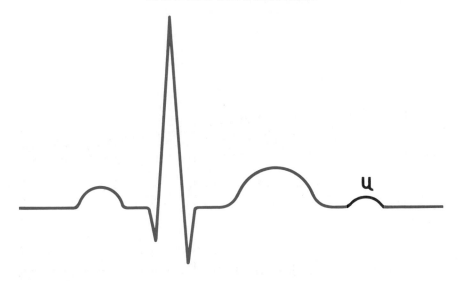

INTERVALS AND SEGMENTS

A point that helps in remembering the measurements we are going to discuss is that intervals contain waves, and segments are the lines between the waves.

PR Interval. The time from the beginning of the P wave to the beginning of the QRS complex is called the *PR interval*. This time interval represents depolarization of the atria and the spread of the depolarization wave up to and including the AV node.

PR Segment. The PR segment represents the period of time between the P wave and the QRS complex.

ST Segment. The distance between the QRS complex and the T wave from the point where the QRS complex ends (J-point) to the onset of the ascending limb of the T wave is called the *ST segment*. On the ECG, this segment is a sensitive indicator of myocardial ischemia or injury.

QT Interval. The time from the beginning of the QRS complex to the end of the T wave is called the *QT interval*. This interval represents both ventricular depolarization and repolarization.

Ventricular Activation Time. The time from the beginning of the QRS complex to the peak of the R wave is called the *ventricular activation time* and represents the time necessary for the depolarization wave to travel from the inner surface of the heart (endocardium) to the outer surface of the heart (epicardium).

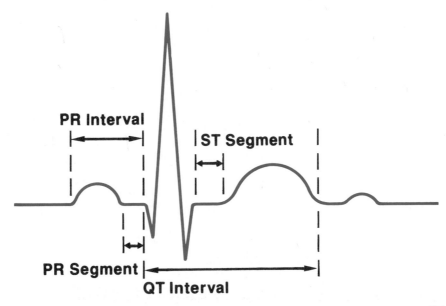

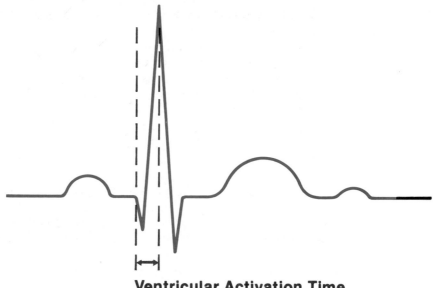

Ventricular Activation Time

KINDS OF QRS COMPLEXES

Our point of reference on the ECG is the isoelectric line. This is the flat line before the P wave or right after the T or U wave. Any stylus movement above this line is considered positive, and any stylus movement below this line is considered negative.

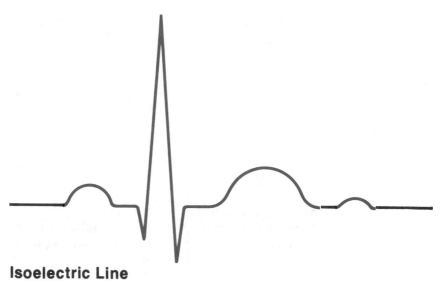

Isoelectric Line

A QRS complex may be composed of a Q wave, R wave, and an S wave, or various combinations thereof.

R wave is a positive deflection.
Q wave is a negative deflection before an R wave.
S wave is a negative deflection after an R wave.

R waves are only positive waves and Q and S waves are only negative waves. We always call a ventricular depolarization complex a QRS complex whether all three waves are present or not.

It is possible to have more than one positive wave in a QRS complex. These positive waves can only be R waves, and to differentiate between the two R waves the second R wave is labeled R prime (R′). The repetition of an S wave is designated by the use of S prime (S′).

DIFFERENT KINDS OF QRS COMPLEXES

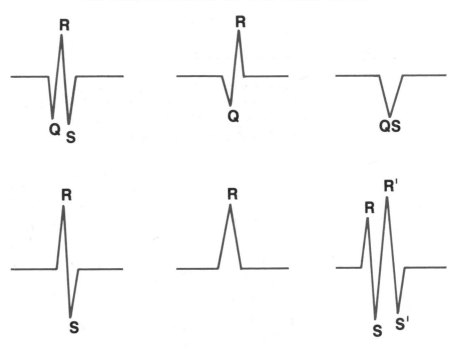

An R wave is a positive deflection.
A Q wave is a negative deflection before an R wave.
An S wave is a negative deflection after an R wave.

PQRSTU WAVES, COMPLEXES, INTERVALS, AND SEGMENTS

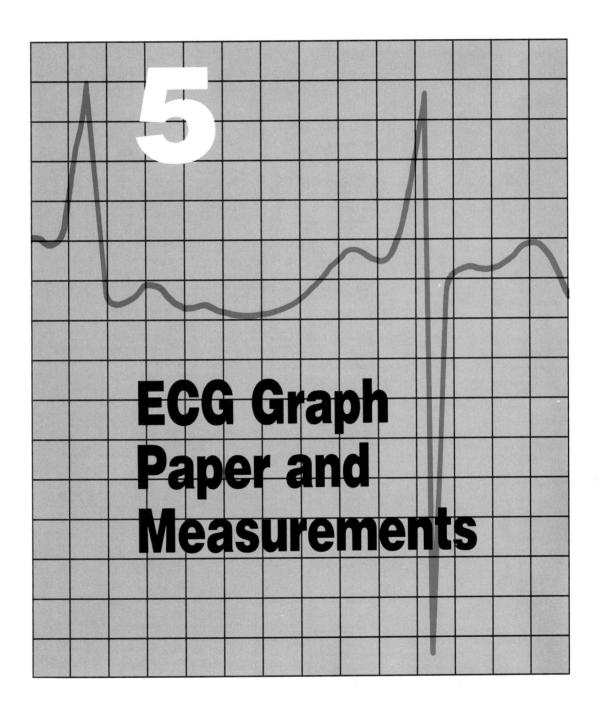

5

ECG Graph Paper and Measurements

TIME AND VOLTAGE

Before understanding the important measurements of the PQRSTU complex, you should become familiar with the ECG graph paper.

On the vertical axis we measure voltage or height in millimeters (mm). Each small square is 1 mm high and each large square is 5 mm high. The isoelectric line is always our reference point.

VOLTAGE

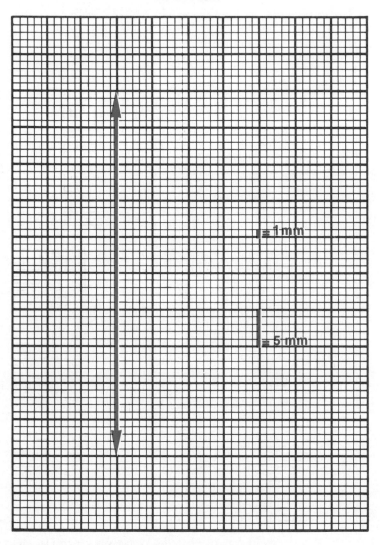

R waves are measured from the top of the isoelectric line to the top point of the R wave. Q and S waves are measured from the bottom of the isoelectric line to the bottom point of the Q or S wave. ST elevation is measured from the top of the isoelectric line to the ST segment, and ST depression is measured from the bottom of the isoelectric line to the ST segment.

VOLTAGE MEASUREMENTS

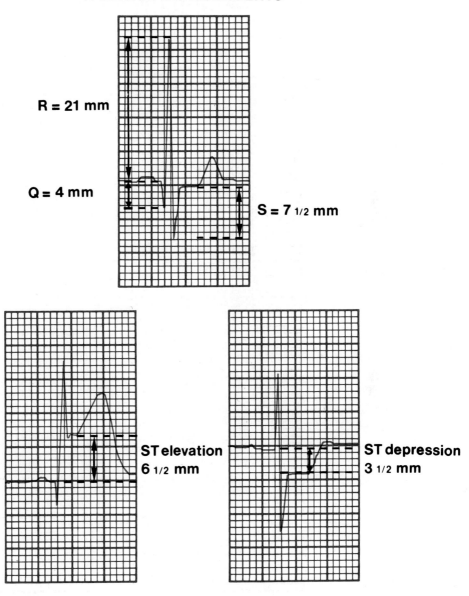

R = 21 mm

Q = 4 mm

S = 7 1/2 mm

ST elevation 6 1/2 mm

ST depression 3 1/2 mm

ECG GRAPH PAPER AND MEASUREMENTS

On the horizontal axis we measure time in seconds. Each small square is .04 second in duration and each large square is .20 second in duration. Five large squares = 1 second (5 × .20).

TIME IN SECONDS

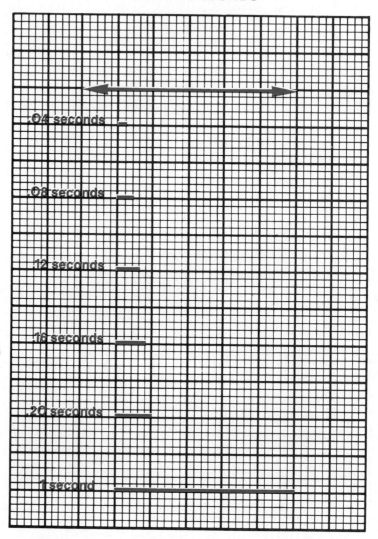

MEASUREMENTS

During our ECG analysis we will be measuring and examining the PR and QRS intervals.

PR Interval. Atrial depolarization and AV conduction time are represented by the PR interval. Measure from the beginning of the P wave, where the P wave lifts off the isoelectric line, to the beginning of the first wave of the QRS complex. Count along the horizontal axis every .04 second (.04, .08, .12, .16, and .20, etc.) until you obtain the correct distance between the two points; this is the PR interval in seconds. The normal range for a PR interval is .12 to .20 second. If the rate of conduction of the sinus impulse through the AV node is faster than .12 second in duration, the term *accelerated conduction* is used. If the rate of conduction of the sinus impulse through the AV node is slower than .20 second, then *first degree AV block* is present.

PR MEASUREMENTS

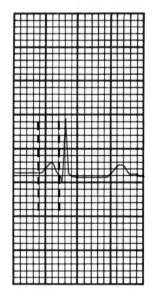 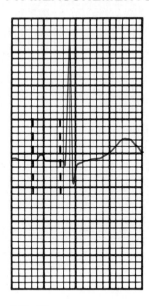 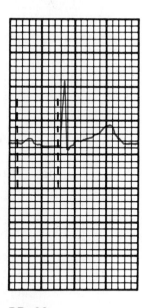

PR .12
Accelerated
AV conduction

PR .18

PR .26
First degree
AV block

QRS Interval. Ventricular depolarization is represented by the QRS interval. Measure from the beginning of the first wave of the QRS where it lifts off the isoelectric line, to the end of the last wave of the QRS where it meets the isoelectric line. Count along the horizontal axis every .04 second until you obtain the distance between the two points; this is the QRS interval in seconds. The normal range for a QRS interval is .04 to .11 second.

QRS MEASUREMENTS

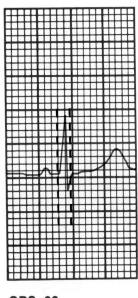 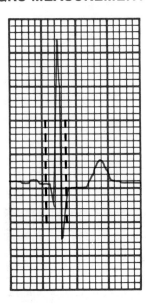 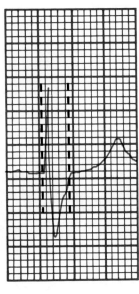

QRS .06   QRS .10   QRS .16

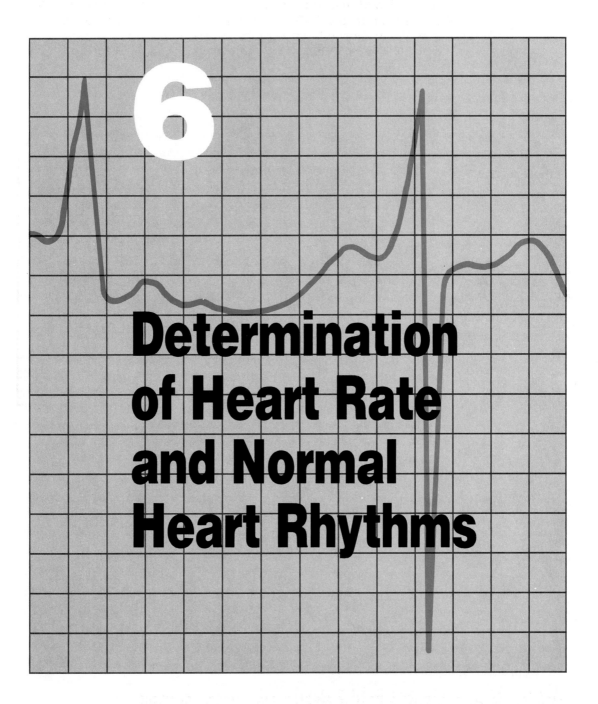

6

Determination of Heart Rate and Normal Heart Rhythms

DETERMINATION OF HEART RATE

Heart rate is the number of heartbeats occurring in 1 minute. On an ECG, the heart rate is measured from R wave to R wave to determine the ventricular rate, and P wave to P wave to determine the atrial rate. Remember, QRS complexes represent ventricular depolarizations and P waves represent atrial depolarizations. In the ECGs presented for interpretation in the following chapters, both the atrial and ventricular rates will be identical.

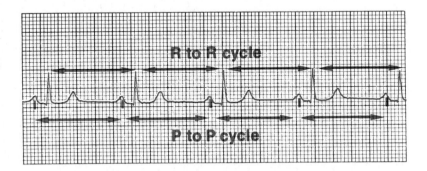

Two methods of calculating heart rate will be demonstrated:

1. **300-150-100-75-60-50.** This method is the easiest and quickest for rate determination. Choose an R wave that falls on or close to a heavy black line on the ECG paper. The first heavy black line to the right is the *300* line, the second is the *150* line, the third is the *100* line, the fourth is the *75* line, the fifth is the *60* line, and the sixth is the *50* line. If the next R wave falls on the fourth heavy black line to the right, the heart rate is 75 beats per minute.

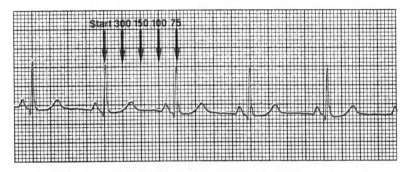

The heart rate is slightly above the rate of 75 beats per minute.

2. **Duration between R waves.** Count the duration in seconds between two R waves and divide this number into 60; this number is the heart rate.

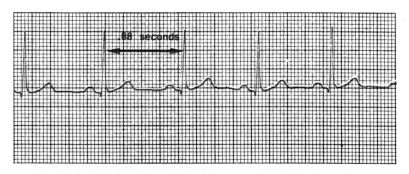

60 divided by .88 seconds = 68 beats per minute

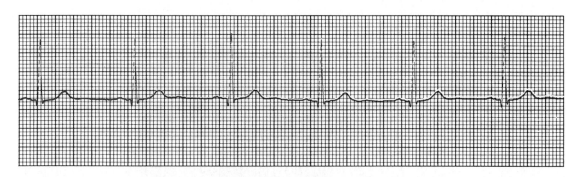

The heart rate is approximately 60 beats per minute.

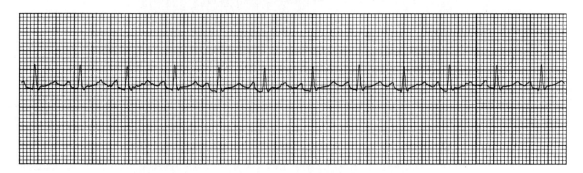

The heart rate is approximately 120 beats per minute.

DETERMINATION OF HEART RATE AND NORMAL HEART RHYTHMS

A normal heart rhythm begins in the SA node and proceeds to depolarize the atria; then a P wave is inscribed on the ECG, representing atrial depolarization. The cardiac impulse travels to the AV node and the bundle of His, transverses the bundle branches and the Purkinje fibers, and a PR interval is recorded. The impulse then reaches the ventricular muscle, and a QRS is displayed representing ventricular depolarization, which is followed by an isoelectric ST segment and a T wave representing ventricular repolarization. This heart rhythm is called *sinus rhythm*. The sinus rhythms are distinguished from one another by rate.

Sinus rhythm—60–100 beats per minute
Sinus bradycardia—below 60 beats per minute
Sinus tachycardia—above 100 beats per minute

CONDUCTION IN SINUS RHYTHM

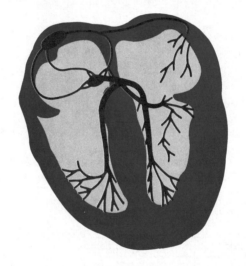

SINUS RHYTHMS

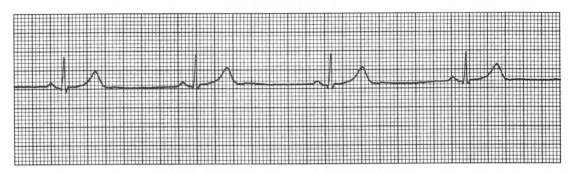

Sinus bradycardia at 43 beats per minute

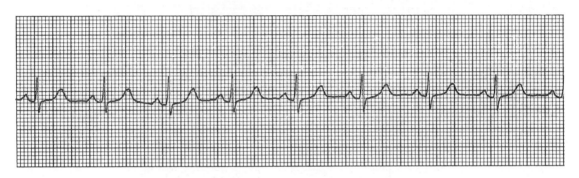

Sinus rhythm at 82 beats per minute

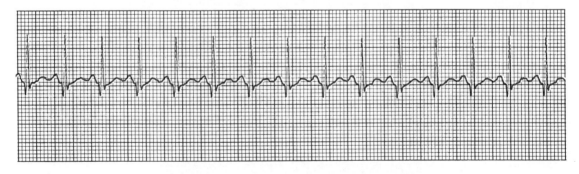

Sinus tachycardia at 149 beats per minute

DETERMINATION OF HEART RATE AND NORMAL HEART RHYTHMS

Sinus arrhythmia is a rhythm beginning in the SA node that demonstrates an irregular rate. This is commonly found in children and young adults and is considered normal. The PP and the RR cycles vary more than .16 second.

SINUS ARRHYTHMIA

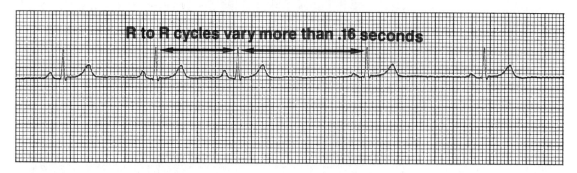

RESPIRATORY SINUS ARRHYTHMIA

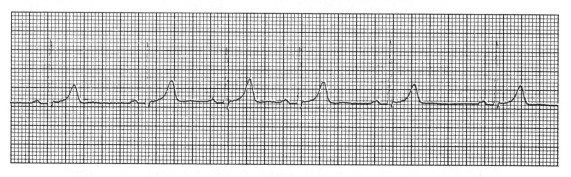

Heart rate increases with inspiration and decreases with expiration.

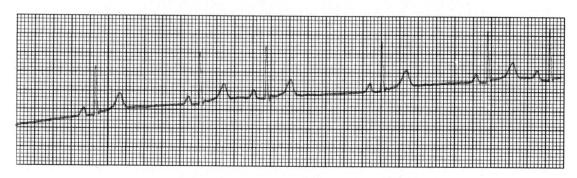

Heart rate varies with respiration in a young adult.

PRACTICE ECG 1

Rate:

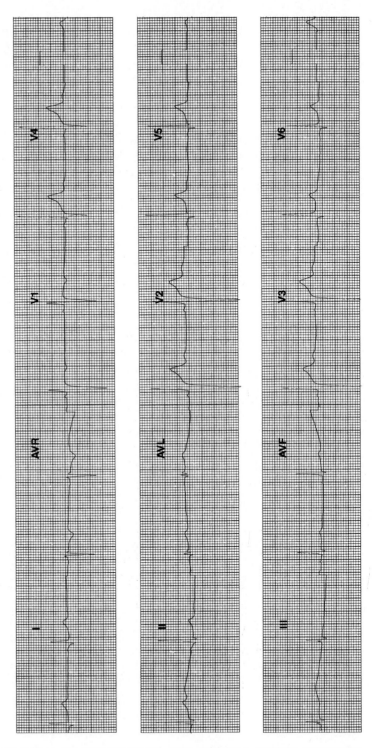

DETERMINATION OF HEART RATE AND NORMAL HEART RHYTHMS

PRACTICE ECG 2

Rate:

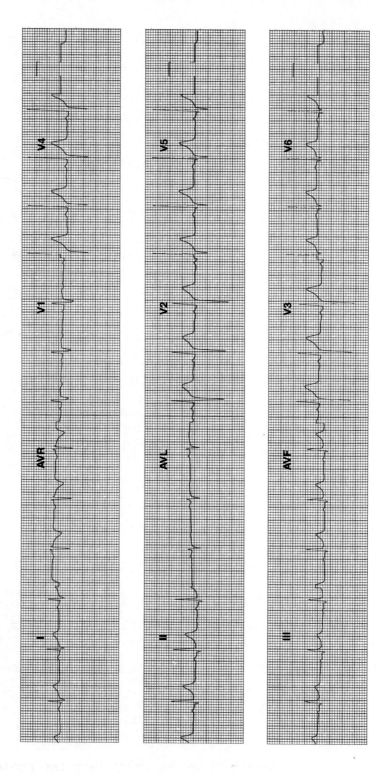

PRACTICE ECG 3

Rate: _____

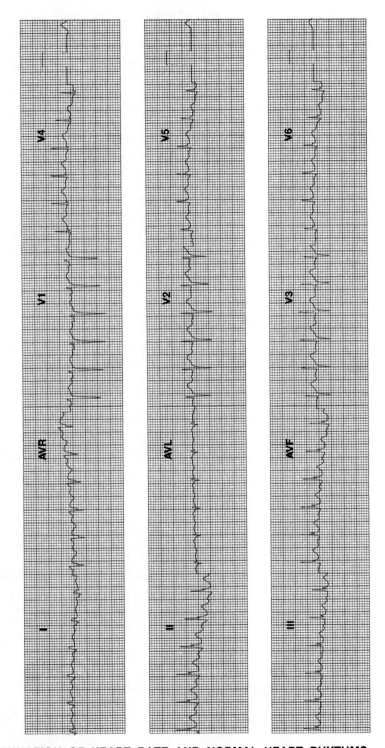

DETERMINATION OF HEART RATE AND NORMAL HEART RHYTHMS

45

PRACTICE ECG 4

Rate:

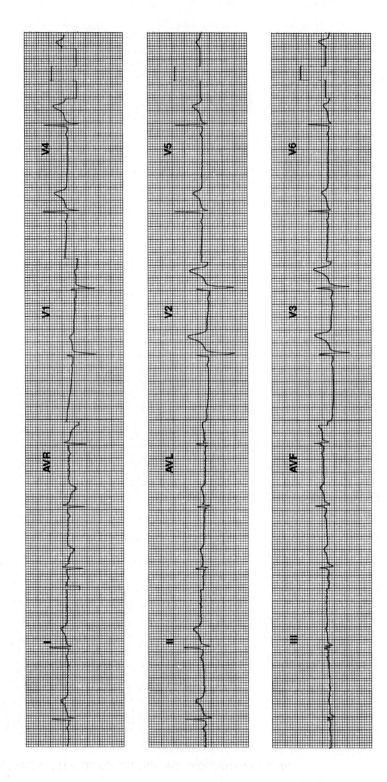

PRACTICE ECG 5

Rate:

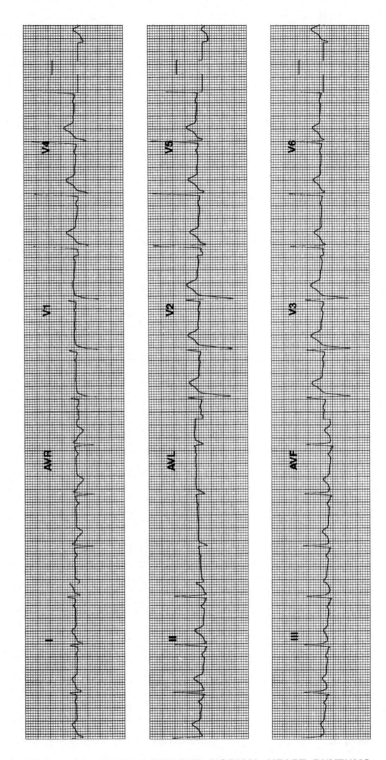

DETERMINATION OF HEART RATE AND NORMAL HEART RHYTHMS

PRACTICE ECG 6

Rate: _____

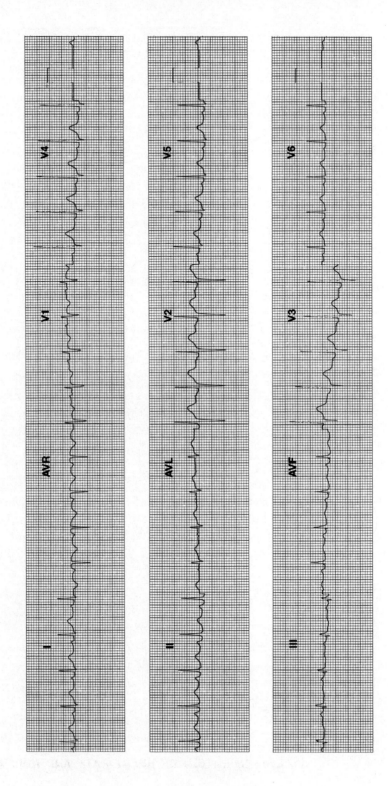

PRACTICE ECG 7

Rate:

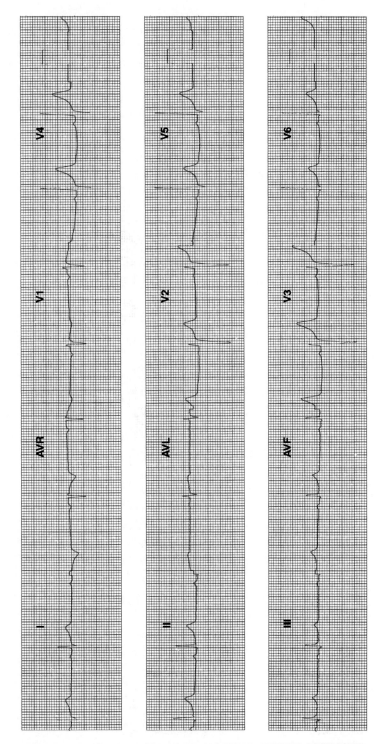

DETERMINATION OF HEART RATE AND NORMAL HEART RHYTHMS

PRACTICE ECG 8

Rate:

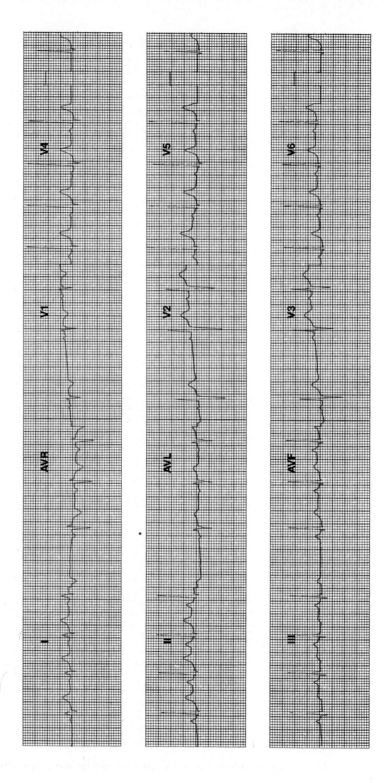

PRACTICE ECG 9

Rate:

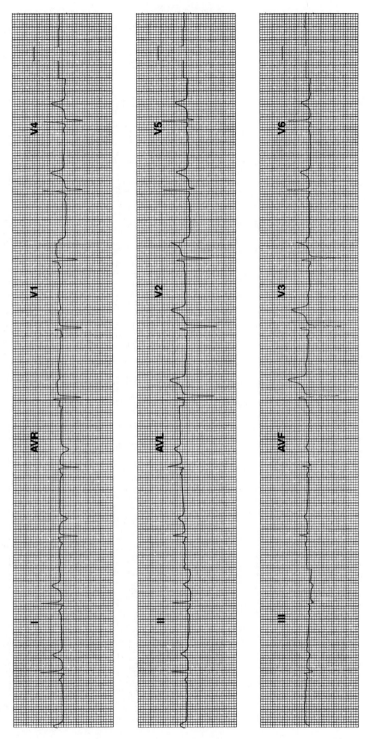

DETERMINATION OF HEART RATE AND NORMAL HEART RHYTHMS

PRACTICE ECG 10

Rate:

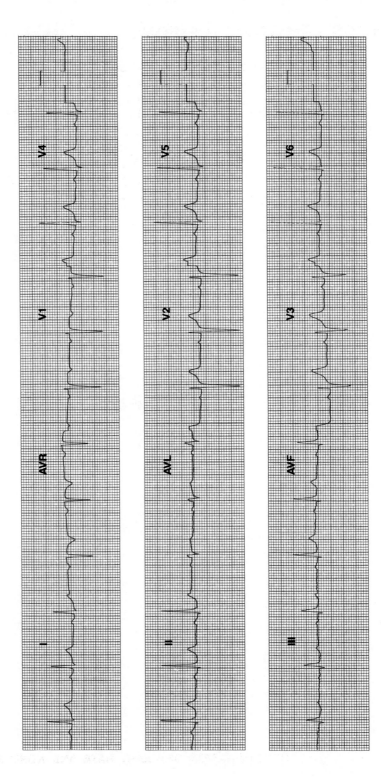

ANSWERS FOR PRACTICE ECGS

1. Sinus bradycardia at 46 beats per minute
2. Sinus rhythm at 79 beats per minute
3. Sinus tachycardia at 140 beats per minute
4. Sinus arrhythmia ranging between 40 and 60 beats per minute
5. Sinus rhythm at 75 beats per minute
6. Sinus tachycardia at 110 beats per minute
7. Sinus bradycardia at 52 beats per minute
8. Sinus arrhythmia ranging between 55 and 90 beats per minute
9. Sinus bradycardia at 55 beats per minute
10. Sinus rhythm at 70 beats per minute

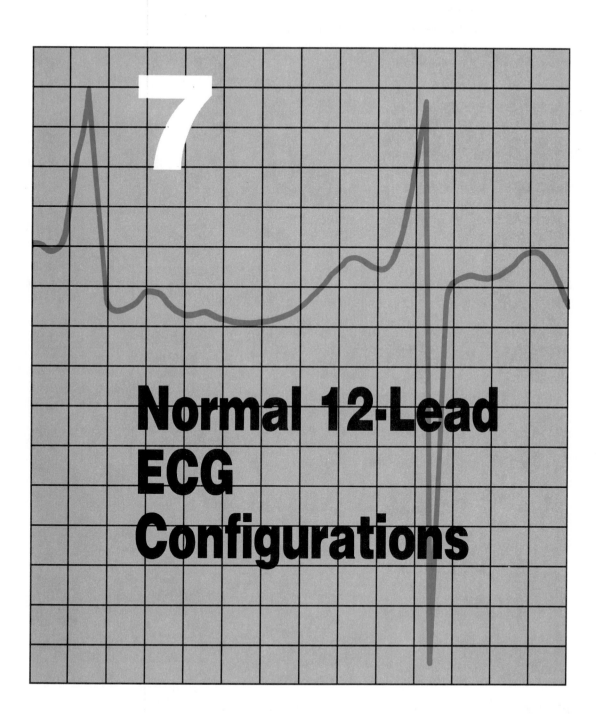

7

Normal 12-Lead ECG Configurations

VECTORS

Each of the 12 ECG leads views the heart from a different angle, so each ECG lead has a separate and sometimes distinct pattern. The standard and augmented leads view the heart in the frontal plane from six different positions, and the six precordial leads examine the heart in the horizontal plane. To demonstrate the configuration of each of the 12 ECG leads, we will show how the wave of depolarization travels within the heart by the use of a vector. A vector illustrates magnitude and direction of the depolarization waves within the heart. A mean QRS vector reveals an average of the depolarization waves in one portion of the heart (*e.g.,* the mean P vector representing atrial depolarization or the mean QRS vector denoting ventricular depolarization).

Let's review the electrical conduction system of the heart, consider the direction of depolarization within the atria and the ventricles, and label the system with vectors. The electrical impulse begins in the SA node and travels to both atria and depolarizes them. The initial wave of atrial depolarization spreads anteriorly through the right atrium and toward the AV node. The next waves of atrial depolarization travel posteriorly and toward the left atrium.

VECTORS

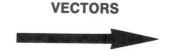

A vector points in the direction of depolarization.

ATRIAL DEPOLARIZATION

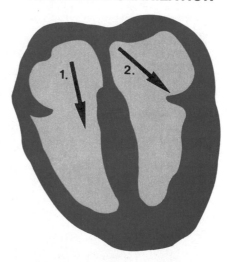

1. **Mean P vector for right atrium**
2. **Mean P vector for left atrium**

A mean P wave vector can be derived that represents the average direction and magnitude of depolarization through both atria. This will point downward and to the patient's left.

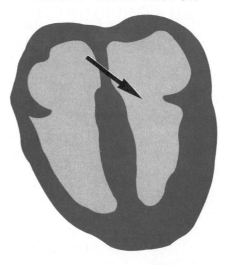

The mean P wave vector, which represents the average of right and left atrial depolarization, will point downward and to the patient's left.

A WAVE OF DEPOLARIZATION MOVING TOWARD AN ELECTRODE WILL RECORD A POSITIVE DEFLECTION ON AN ECG.

A WAVE OF DEPOLARIZATION TRAVELING AWAY FROM AN ELECTRODE WILL INSCRIBE A NEGATIVE DEFLECTION ON AN ECG.

A WAVE OF DEPOLARIZATION MOVING AT RIGHT ANGLES TO AN ELECTRODE WILL CAUSE EITHER NO DEFLECTION OR A VERY SMALL DEFLECTION ON AN ECG.

NORMAL 12-LEAD ECG CONFIGURATIONS

STANDARD, AUGMENTED, AND PRECORDIAL LEAD CONFIGURATIONS

The wave of atrial depolarization is moving downward and to the patient's left, directly toward lead II on an ECG. Lead II will record the tallest P wave. The wave of atrial depolarization is moving away from lead aVR so a negative P wave will be inscribed in this lead. The wave of atrial depolarization is moving at approximately right angles to lead III or aVL, so the smallest P wave will be seen in these leads.

MEAN P WAVE VECTOR

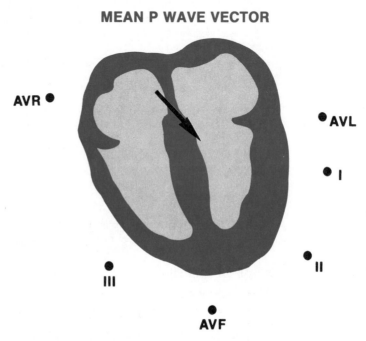

Lead II will have the tallest P wave because the mean P wave vector is moving directly toward it.

Lead aVR will have a negative P wave because the mean P wave vector is moving directly away from it.

Lead III or Lead aVL will have the smallest P wave because the mean P wave vector is moving at approximately right angles to it.

The P wave should always be positive in lead II and not wider than .11 second or taller than 2.4 mm. Lead aVR should always have an inverted P wave.

NORMAL P WAVE CONFIGURATIONS

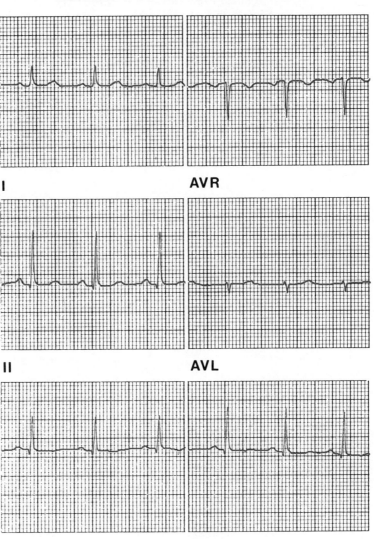

I

AVR

II

AVL

III

AVF

The P wave is most positive in II.
The P wave is negative in aVR.
The P wave is smallest in III or aVL.

NORMAL 12-LEAD ECG CONFIGURATIONS

After atrial depolarization, the wave of depolarization travels to the ventricles by way of the AV node, bundle of His, and the bundle branches. We will divide ventricular depolarization into three main stages, each represented by a vector:

Vector 1. Septal activation and early right ventricular depolarization—the first activation in the ventricles occurs in the septum as it is depolarized from left to right. Early depolarization of the right ventricle also occurs.

VECTOR 1

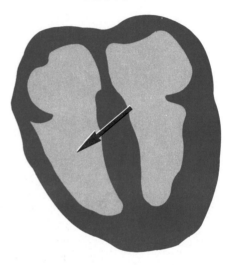

Septal and early right ventricular activation

Vector 2. Apical activation—the second major ventricular activation is the depolarization of the right and left ventricular apex and the completion of right ventricular depolarization.

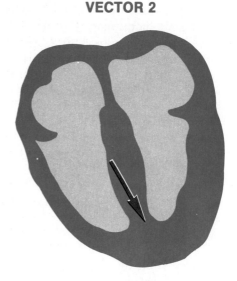

Apical activation

Vector 3. Left ventricular activation—the remainder of the left ventricle is depolarized toward the lateral wall. Because the right ventricle has already completed depolarization, the left ventricle will depolarize unopposed by the right, so large voltages will be inscribed at this time.

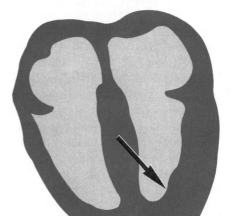

Left ventricular activation

NORMAL 12-LEAD ECG CONFIGURATIONS

If we place the six frontal and six precordial ECG leads on a diagram of the heart that depicts the three main stages of ventricular depolarization, you can easily see how each of the 12 ECG leads is derived. Vector 1, representing septal and early right ventricular activation, is moving away from all of the leads on the left side of the heart, so an initial negative deflection will be inscribed in the form of a Q wave. Leads on the right side of the heart will have the initial vector moving toward them, so an initial positive deflection will be recorded in the form of an R wave. The leads at the bottom of the heart that are at approximately right angles to the initial vector will demonstrate either no deflection or a very small deflection at this time.

Vector 2 represents the second major force of ventricular depolarization, labeled *apical activation,* and is moving approximately toward the ECG leads on the left side of the heart and at the bottom of the heart. A positive deflection in the form of an R wave will be recorded in the left heart leads, and because the vector is moving predominantly away from the right heart leads, a negative deflection or an S wave will be recorded.

Vector 3 illustrates the forces of left ventricular activation. The right ventricle has already depolarized, so the left ventricle will depolarize unopposed by the right and will display large positive voltages in the left heart leads as the electrical forces are moving toward them, and large negative voltages in the form of S waves in the right heart leads as the forces are moving away from them.

THE THREE STAGES OF VENTRICULAR DEPOLARIZATION

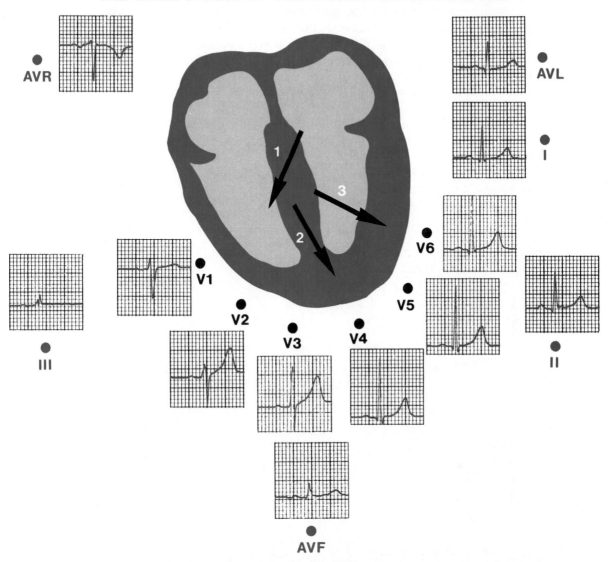

A wave of depolarization moving toward an electrode will record a positive deflection on an ECG.

A wave of depolarization traveling away from an electrode will inscribe a negative deflection on an ECG.

A wave of depolarization moving at right angles to an electrode will cause either no deflection or a very small deflection on an ECG.

NORMAL 12-LEAD ECG CONFIGURATIONS

Although the limb leads are open to some variability in their configuration, the chest leads must remain within a more standard format to be considered normal. The QRS should have a small R wave and a larger S wave in V_1, with the R wave becoming progressively larger and the S wave becoming progressively smaller or nonexistent when it reaches V_6. The area of transition where the R wave becomes equal to or larger than the S wave should occur in V_3 or V_4.

If the transition occurs in V_1 or V_2 it is considered an *early transition*, and if it occurs in V_5 or V_6 it is considered a *late transition*.

PRECORDIAL LEAD CONFIGURATIONS

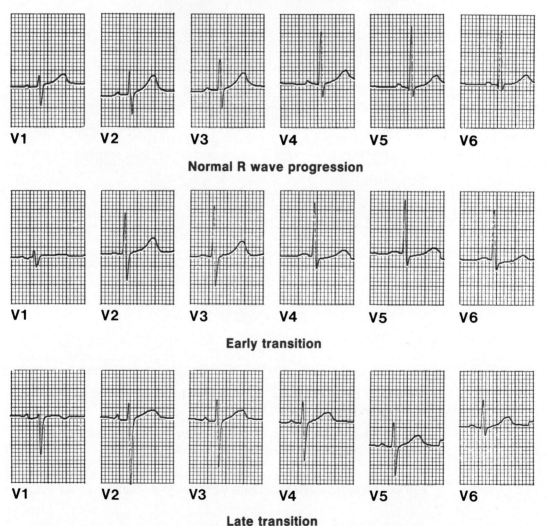

Normal R wave progression

Early transition

Late transition

HOW TO QUICKLY AND ACCURATELY MASTER ECG INTERPRETATION

A mean QRS vector can be derived that represents the average direction and magnitude of depolarization through both ventricles. This will point downward and to the patient's left, somewhere in the bottom quarter of the heart. Leads falling in this section of the heart will be predominantly positive because the mean QRS vector is moving toward them, and the leads falling outside this segment will have various combinations, depending on their exact location.

MEAN QRS VECTOR

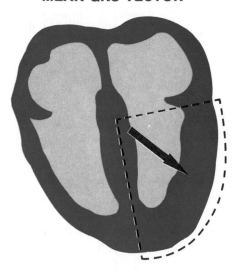

Ventricular repolarization is represented by the T wave and immediately follows ventricular depolarization. The T wave should be upright in leads I, II, aVL, aVF, and V_2–V_6, variable in leads III and V_1, and inverted in lead aVR. If a U wave is present, it should be in the same direction as the T wave. The ST segment should be isoelectric, not varying more than 1 mm above or below the isoelectric line.

NORMAL T WAVE CONFIGURATIONS ON 12-LEAD ECG

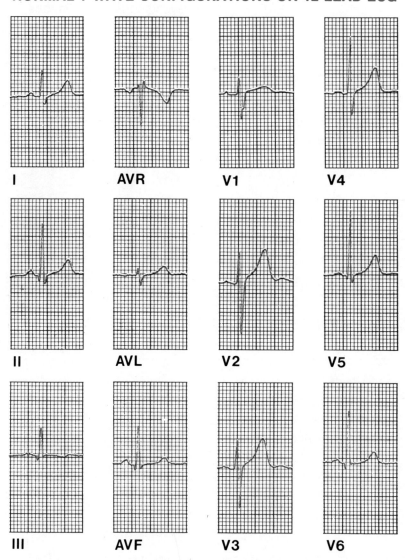

T waves should be upright in leads, I, II, aVL, aVF, V_2–V_6, and inverted in aVR. T waves are variable in leads III and V_1.

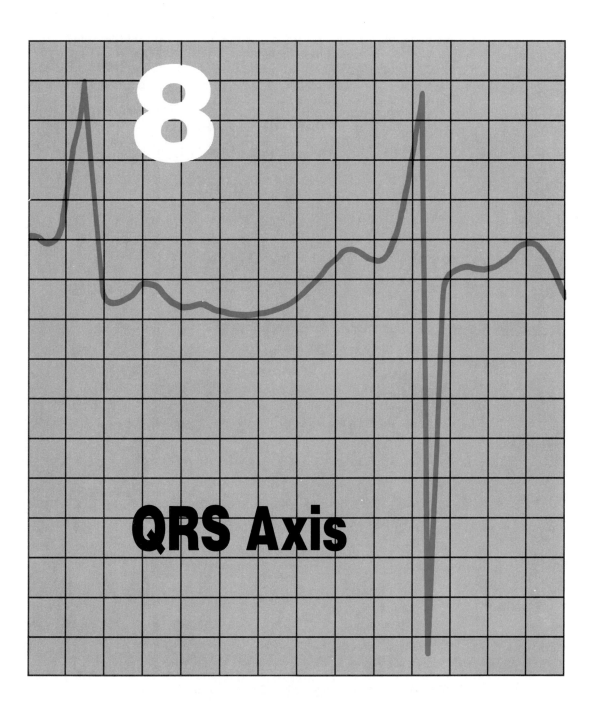

8

QRS Axis

HEXAXIAL REFERENCE SYSTEM

The QRS axis indicates the direction of the mean QRS vector within the heart. It refers to the average direction of depolarization that spreads through the ventricles. The QRS axis can be determined by using the hexaxial reference system. This system is formulated by placing the six frontal plane leads of an ECG around the heart in their respective ECG lead positions and by their positive poles. (See Chapter 1 if a review of this concept is needed.)

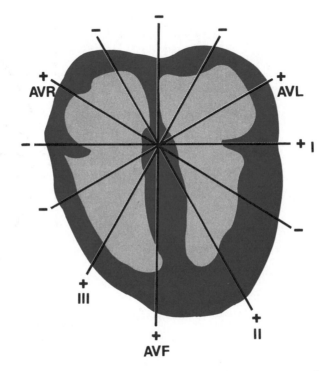

The six ECG limb leads are placed around the heart in their respective ECG lead positions by their positive poles.

The heart is divided, as if a circle, into segments each separated by 30°. Lead I's positive pole is at 0° and proceeding clockwise every division is at 30° increments in a positive category. Going in a counterclockwise direction from lead I, every division is in 30° increments in a minus category.

HEXAXIAL REFERENCE SYSTEM

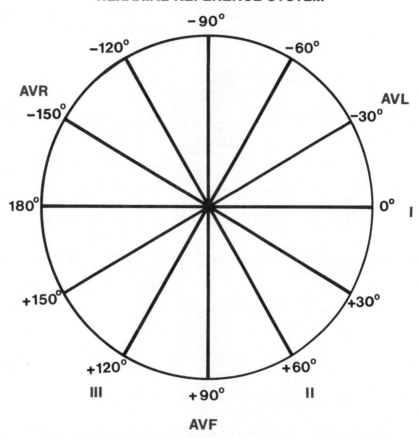

The axis is calculated using the hexaxial reference system.

A normal axis is from 0° to +90°. A left axis is from −1° to −90° and a right axis is from +91° to +180°. The last segment of the circle that is left undesignated is from −179° to −91°. This portion can be considered to be either extreme left or extreme right axis deviation.

AXIS

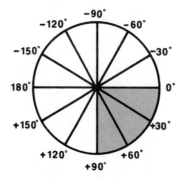

normal axis

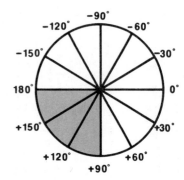

right axis

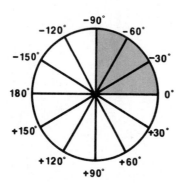

left axis

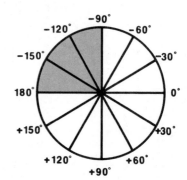

extreme right or left axis

AXIS DETERMINATION

There are three quick and easy ways to calculate the QRS axis on an ECG using leads I, II, III, aVR, aVL, and aVF:

1. The tallest QRS is found in the ECG lead that points directly toward the QRS axis.
2. The most negative QRS is seen in the ECG lead that points directly away from the QRS axis.
3. An equiphasic QRS (a positive and negative wave of the same voltage) is in the ECG lead that is at right angles to the QRS axis.

To begin axis determination, first look at the six frontal plane leads on your ECG and find the lead in which the QRS has the most voltage, either positive or negative. If the most voltage is positive (R wave), it points directly toward the axis. If the most voltage is negative (Q or S wave) it points directly away from the axis. If the most voltage is found in lead II and the voltage is positive, then the QRS axis will point directly toward that lead and the axis will be +60°. If the most voltage on an ECG is found in lead III, but the voltage is negative, then the QRS axis will point directly away from this lead and the axis will be −60°.

AXIS CALCULATIONS USING THE QRS COMPLEX WITH THE MOST VOLTAGE

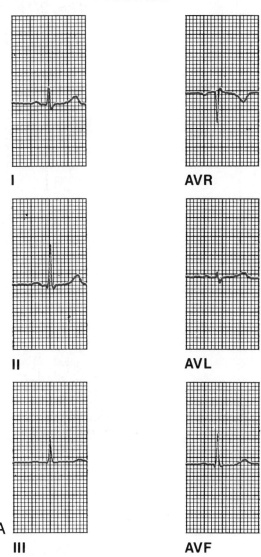

The QRS in lead II has the most voltage. The voltage is positive so the mean QRS vector is pointing directly toward lead II or at +60°. Axis = +60°.

QRS AXIS

AXIS CALCULATIONS USING THE QRS COMPLEX WITH THE MOST VOLTAGE

AXIS CALCULATIONS USING THE QRS COMPLEX WITH THE MOST VOLTAGE

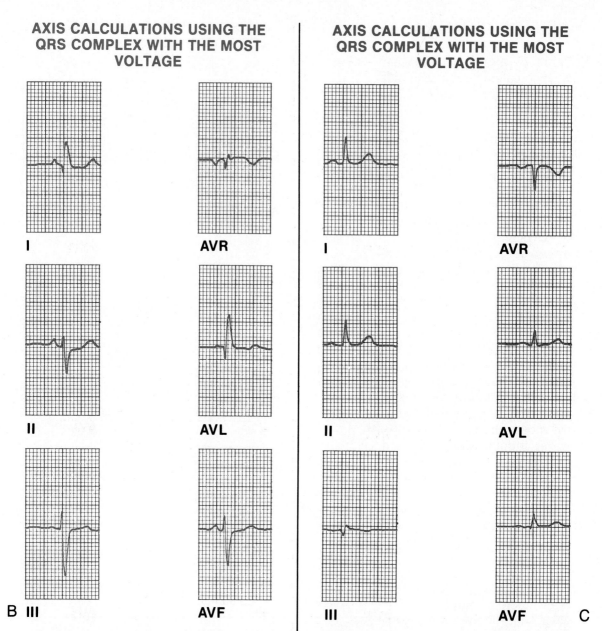

I   AVR

II   AVL

B III   AVF

I   AVR

II   AVL

III   AVF C

The QRS in lead III has the most voltage. The voltage is negative so the mean QRS vector is pointing directly away from lead III or at −60°. Axis = −60°.

The QRS complexes in lead I and lead II have the most voltage. The voltage is equally positive in both leads so the mean QRS vector is pointing directly between lead I and lead II or at +30°. Axis = +30°.

AXIS CALCULATIONS USING THE QRS COMPLEX WITH THE MOST VOLTAGE

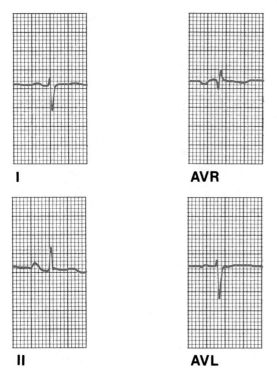

I

AVR

II

AVL

D III

AVF

The QRS in lead III has the most voltage. The voltage is positive so the mean QRS vector is pointing directly toward lead III or at +120°. Axis = +120°.

AXIS CALCULATIONS USING THE QRS COMPLEX WITH THE MOST VOLTAGE

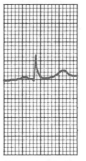
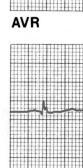

I

AVR

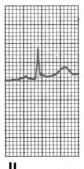
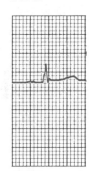

II

AVL

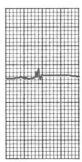

III

AVF E

The QRS complexes in leads II and aVR have the most voltage. The voltage in aVR is negative so the mean QRS vector is pointing directly away from it or at +30°. The voltage in II is positive so the mean QRS vector is pointing directly toward it or at +60°. An average of the two voltages is +45°. Axis = +45°.

If you find an ECG that has an equiphasic QRS in a lead, then that lead is at right angles to the QRS axis. With an equiphasic QRS in lead I, your axis will be at right angles to lead I, either +90° or −90°. One more step is necessary to decide in which direction to proceed. Check lead II on the ECG. If that lead has a predominantly positive QRS, then the QRS axis is in that general direction, which would be +90°. If you check lead II and discover that the QRS is predominantly negative, then you know that the QRS axis is going away from lead II and that the axis would be −90°.

AXIS CALCULATIONS USING EQUIPHASIC QRS COMPLEXES

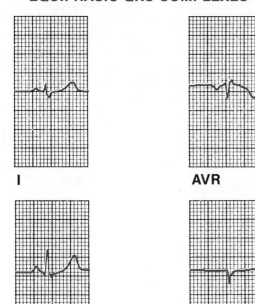

I

AVR

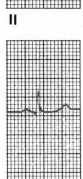

II

AVL

III

AVF

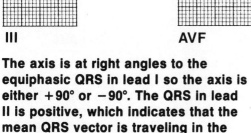

The axis is at right angles to the equiphasic QRS in lead I so the axis is either +90° or −90°. The QRS in lead II is positive, which indicates that the mean QRS vector is traveling in the general direction of +60°. Axis = +90°.

AXIS CALCULATIONS USING EQUIPHASIC QRS COMPLEXES

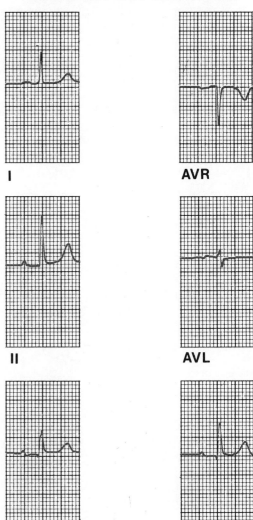

I

AVR

II

AVL

III

AVF

The axis is at a right angle to the equiphasic QRS in lead aVL so the axis is either +60° or −120°. The QRS in II is positive, which indicates that the mean QRS vector is traveling in the general direction of +60°. Axis = +60°.

QRS AXIS

AXIS CALCULATIONS USING EQUIPHASIC QRS COMPLEXES

AXIS CALCULATIONS USING EQUIPHASIC QRS COMPLEXES

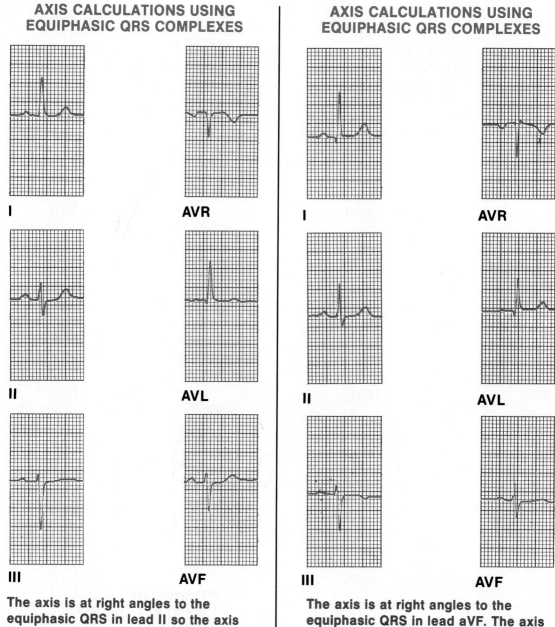

I

AVR

II

AVL

III

AVF

The axis is at right angles to the equiphasic QRS in lead II so the axis is either −30° or +150°. The QRS in III is negative, which indicates that the mean QRS vector is traveling away from +120°. Axis = −30°.

The axis is at right angles to the equiphasic QRS in lead aVF. The axis is either ±180 or 0°. The QRS in II is positive, which indicates that the mean QRS vector is traveling in the general direction of +60°. Axis = 0°.

Occasionally, you will find an ECG in which all of the six frontal plane leads are equiphasic. This arrangement makes it impossible to decide on a correct axis, and so we'll call this an indeterminate axis.

INDETERMINATE AXIS

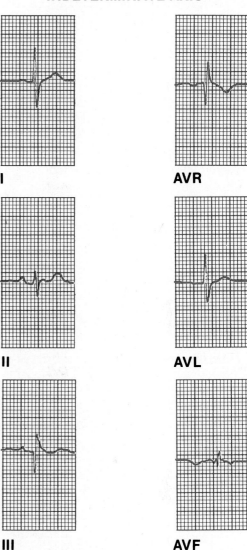

I

AVR

II

AVL

III

AVF

All QRS complexes are equiphasic, which makes axis calculations impossible.

PRACTICE ECG 1

QRS Axis:

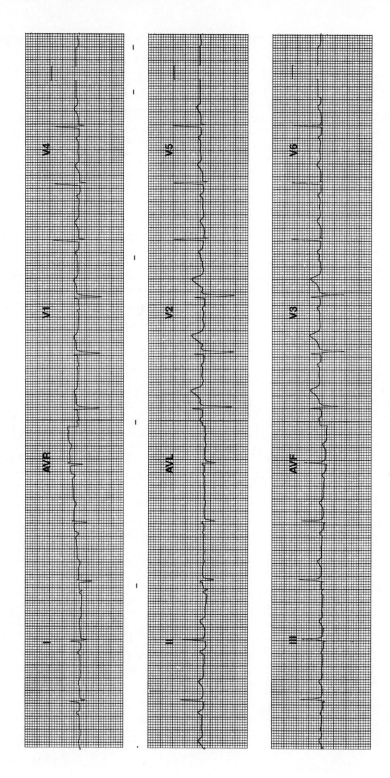

PRACTICE ECG 2

QRS Axis:

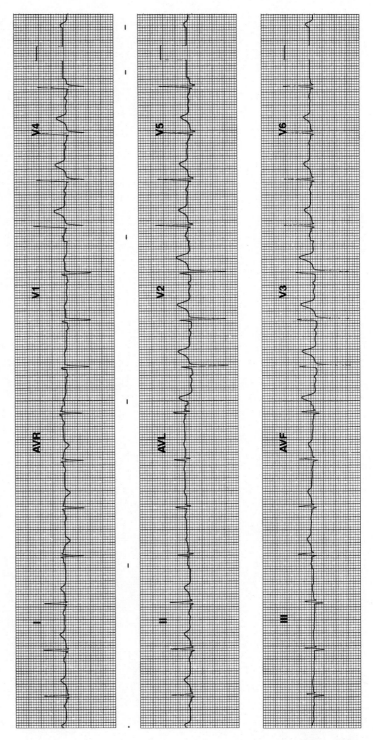

PRACTICE ECG 3

QRS Axis:

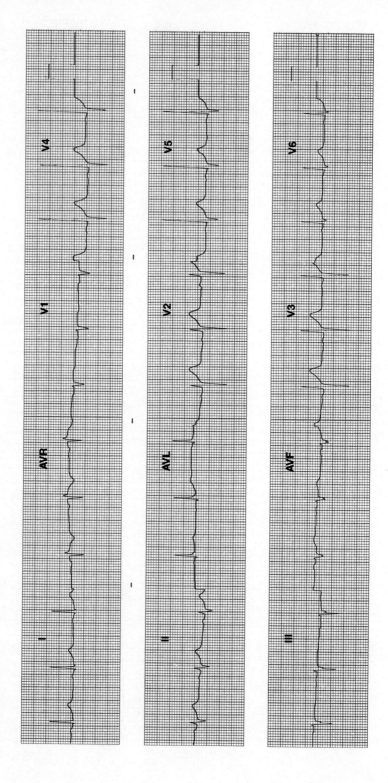

PRACTICE ECG 4

QRS Axis:

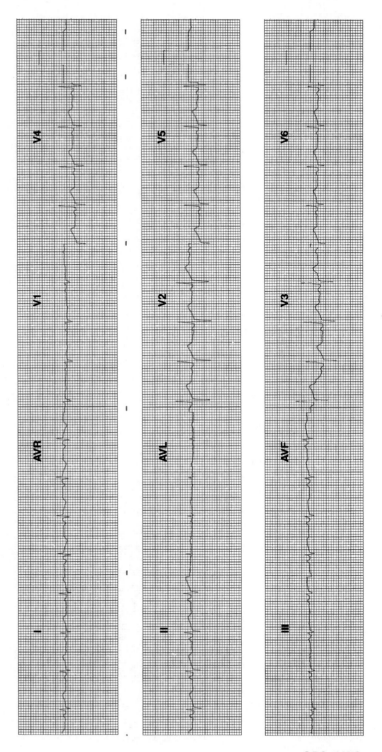

QRS AXIS

PRACTICE ECG 5

QRS Axis:

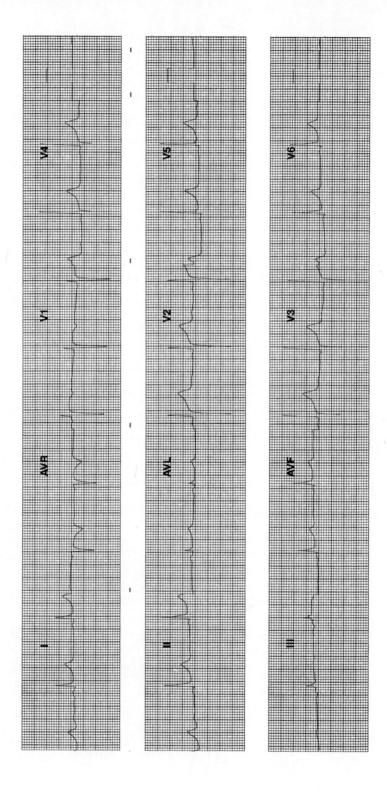

PRACTICE ECG 6

QRS Axis:

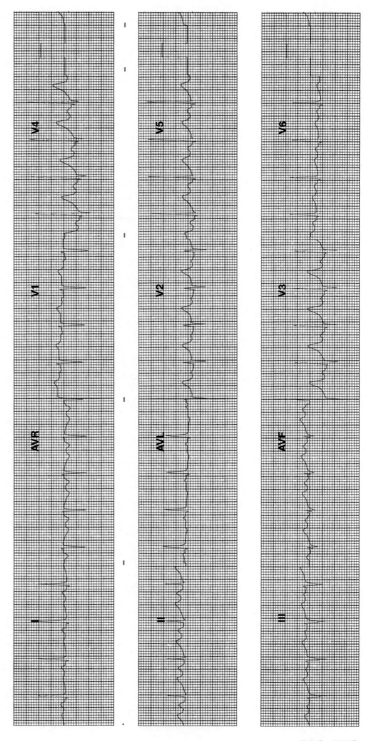

QRS AXIS

PRACTICE ECG 7

QRS Axis:

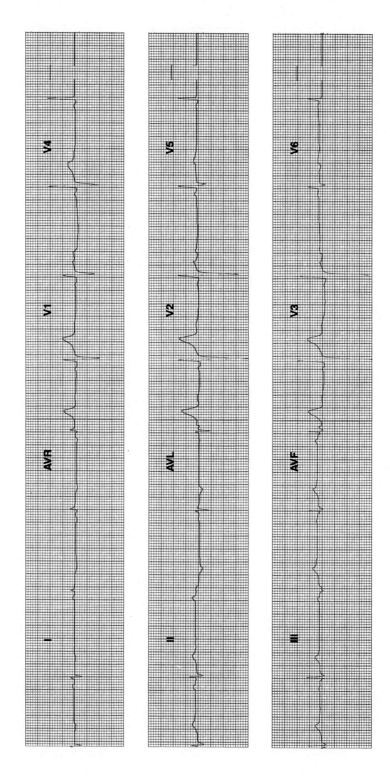

PRACTICE ECG 8

QRS Axis:

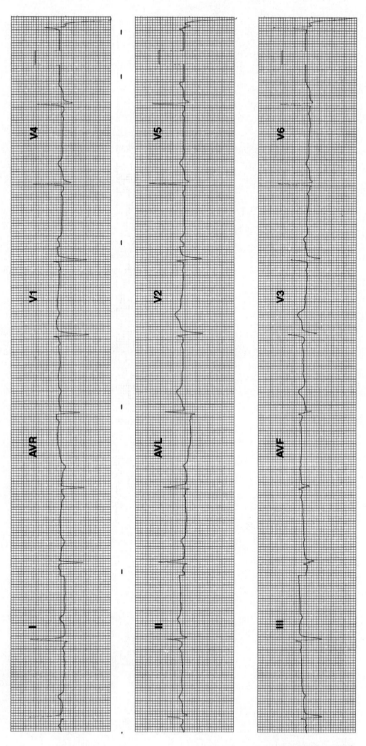

QRS AXIS

PRACTICE ECG 9

QRS Axis:

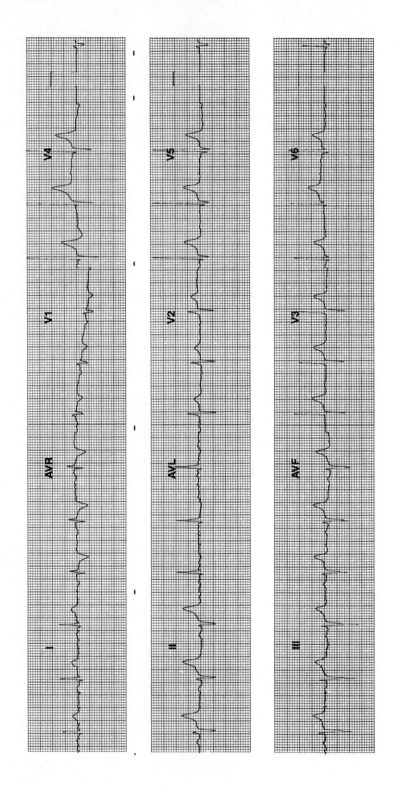

PRACTICE ECG 10

QRS Axis:

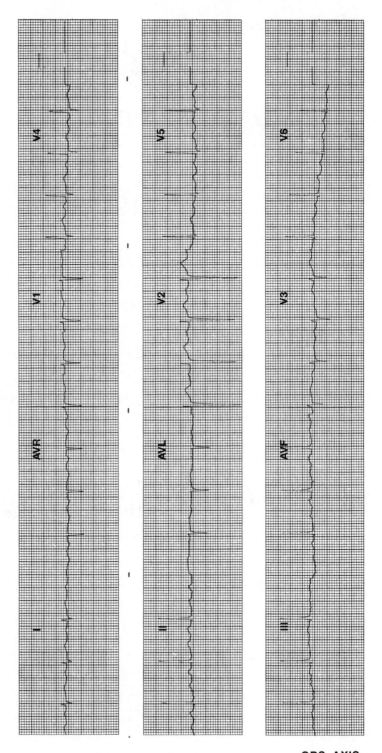

QRS AXIS

ANSWERS FOR PRACTICE ECGS

1. +90° Right axis deviation
2. +30°
3. −30° Left axis deviation
4. Indeterminate axis
5. +60°
6. 0°
7. +120° Right axis deviation
8. 0°
9. −60° Left axis deviation
10. +90° Right axis deviation

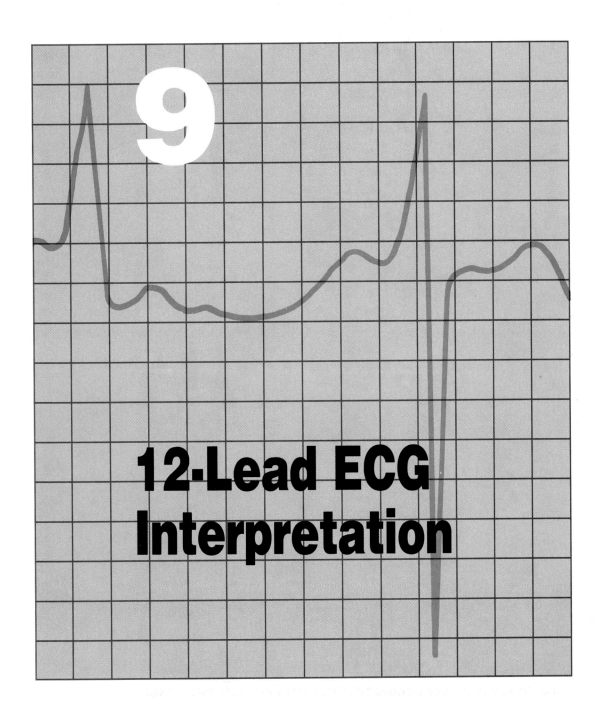

9

12-Lead ECG
Interpretation

TECHNICALLY ACCURATE ECG TRACING

The most important part of ECG interpretation is to begin with a technically accurate tracing. Let's ensure that the ECG has been recorded correctly. Using Einthoven's equation (lead II = lead I + lead III), the voltage in lead II should equal the voltage of both I and III together. The P wave should be positive in lead II and negative in aVR.

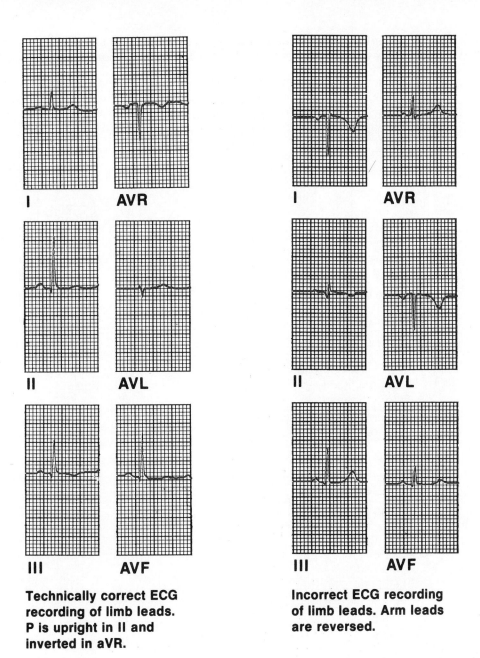

I	AVR
II	AVL
III	AVF

Technically correct ECG recording of limb leads. P is upright in II and inverted in aVR.

I	AVR
II	AVL
III	AVF

Incorrect ECG recording of limb leads. Arm leads are reversed.

In the chest leads, normal R wave progression should be present. The R wave should be small in V_1 and should become progressively larger as it travels to V_6.

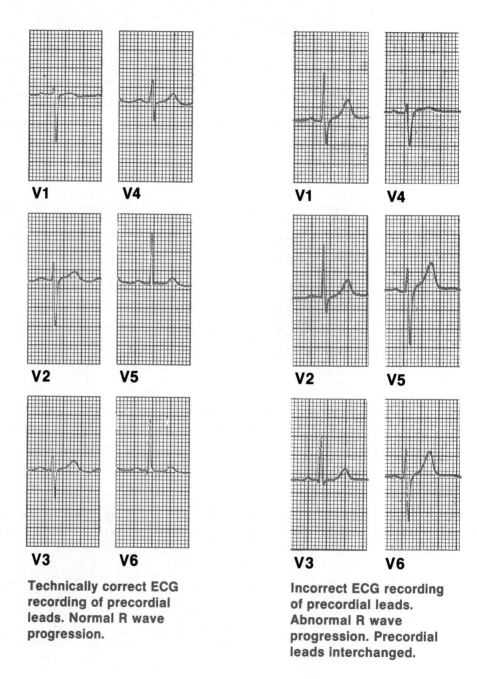

V1	V4
V2	V5
V3	V6

Technically correct ECG recording of precordial leads. Normal R wave progression.

V1	V4
V2	V5
V3	V6

Incorrect ECG recording of precordial leads. Abnormal R wave progression. Precordial leads interchanged.

ARTIFACT

Once we're assured of a technically correct ECG recording we now become concerned with the quality of the tracing. We're looking for an ECG recording that has no outside interference introduced into it and in which the lines making up the waves and intervals are satisfactory. Any outside markings on the ECG represent artifact. The three different types of artifact that are usually encountered are: (1) AC interference, (2) somatic muscle tremor, and (3) wandering baseline.

AC Interference. This artifact originates outside the patient and comes from electrical interference at the patient's bedside.

AC INTERFERENCE

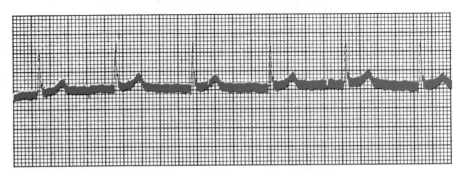

Somatic Muscle Tremor. This artifact is created by the patient himself and usually involves tense muscles or muscle movement.

SOMATIC MUSCLE TREMOR

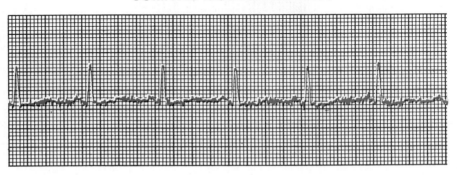

Wandering Baseline. This is caused by poor electrode contact with the patient's skin. Dirty electrodes or insufficient electrode cream can inhibit good contact. The patient's skin may be oily, dirty, scaly, or have an excess amount of body hair, making good electrode contact impossible.

WANDERING BASELINE

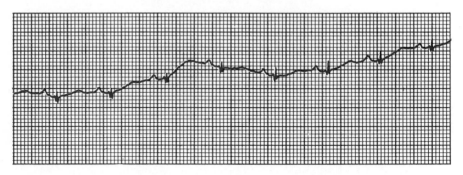

Any one of these artifacts makes the measurement of intervals and assessment of segments and waves extremely difficult, if not impossible.

STANDARDIZATION

To ensure that each ECG tracing is correct as to voltage, the baseline should deflect exactly 10 mm with 1 mV of current. This is called *full*

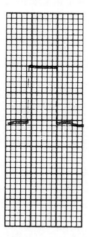

Full standardization

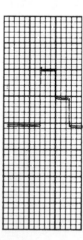

Full standardization limb leads, half standardization precordial leads

standardization. If voltages are extremely large, *half standardization* may be used, which will result in voltages one half their normal size. Often, just the precordial lead voltage is extreme, and it is recorded at half standard while the limb leads are recorded at full standard. These adaptations are demonstrated by means of the standardization or calibration mark. Always check ECG standardization before interpreting an ECG.

12-LEAD ECG INTERPRETATION

Now that we have completed the basic concepts of ECG interpretation, let's put them all together and form a guide to follow for all ECGs that require interpretation in the following chapters:

1. Measure the PR interval in lead II. A normal range is from .12 to .20 second. A PR interval shorter than .12 second is considered accelerated AV conduction, and a PR interval longer than .20 second is first degree AV block.
2. Measure the QRS interval. The normal range is from .04 to .11 second.
3. Calculate the heart rate and rhythm.
4. Calculate the QRS axis.
5. Examine the ST segment for more than 1 mm of elevation or depression.
6. Check the T waves, which should be upright in all leads except aVR, V_1, and possibly III.
7. If no abnormalities are present, the interpretation will be normal ECG.

PRACTICE ECGs—NORMAL ECG INTERPRETATION

Each ECG record demonstrated in this chapter will conform with the following format for interpretation:

PR:
QRS:
QRS axis:
Rate:
Interpretation:

PRACTICE ECG 1

PR:

QRS:

QRS Axis:

Rate:

Interpretation:

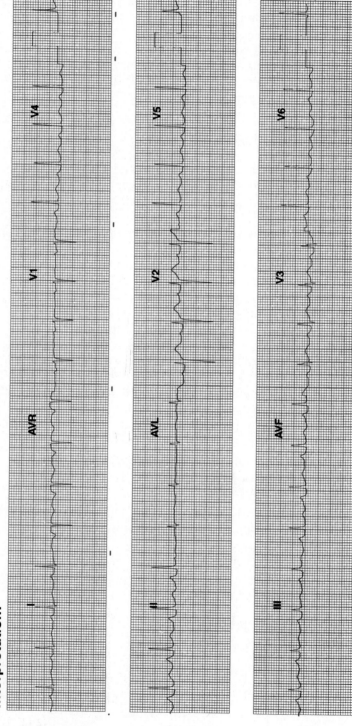

PRACTICE ECG 2

PR:

QRS:

QRS Axis:

Rate:

Interpretation:

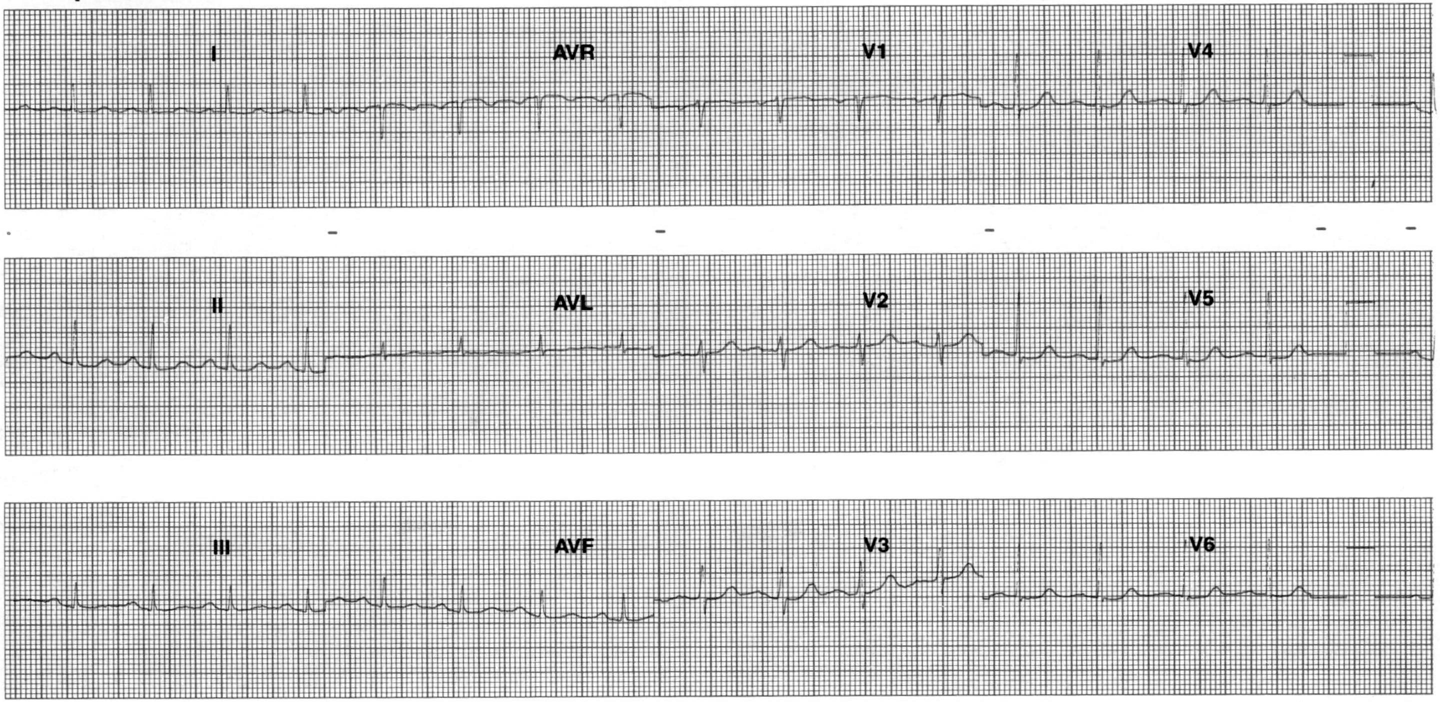

12-LEAD ECG INTERPRETATION

PRACTICE ECG 3

PR:

QRS:

QRS Axis:

Rate:

Interpretation:

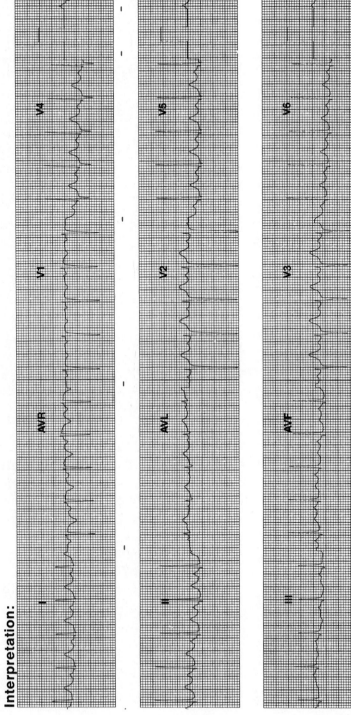

PRACTICE ECG 4

PR:

QRS:

QRS Axis:

Rate:

Interpretation:

12-LEAD ECG INTERPRETATION

PRACTICE ECG 5

PR:

QRS:

QRS Axis:

Rate:

Interpretation:

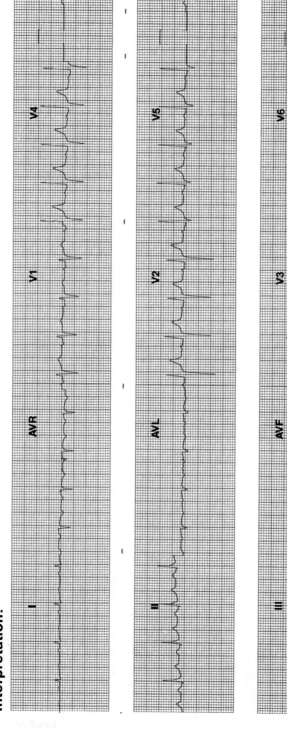

PRACTICE ECG 6

PR:

QRS:

QRS Axis:

Rate:

Interpretation:

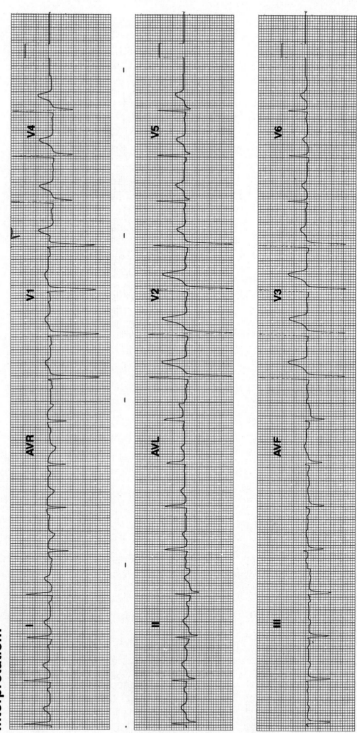

12-LEAD ECG INTERPRETATION

PRACTICE ECG 7

PR:

QRS:

QRS Axis:

Rate:

Interpretation:

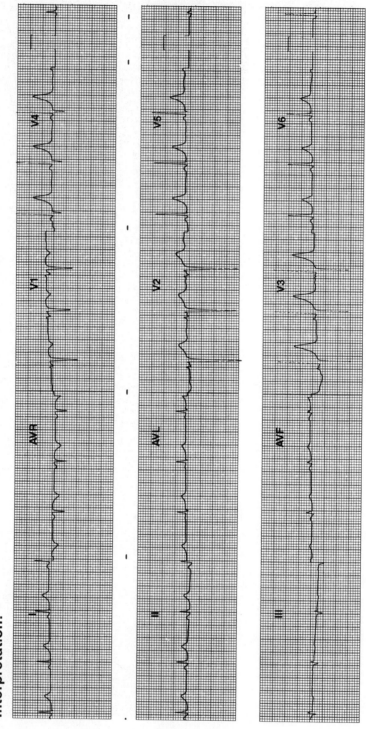

PRACTICE ECG 8

PR:

QRS:

QRS Axis:

Rate:

Interpretation:

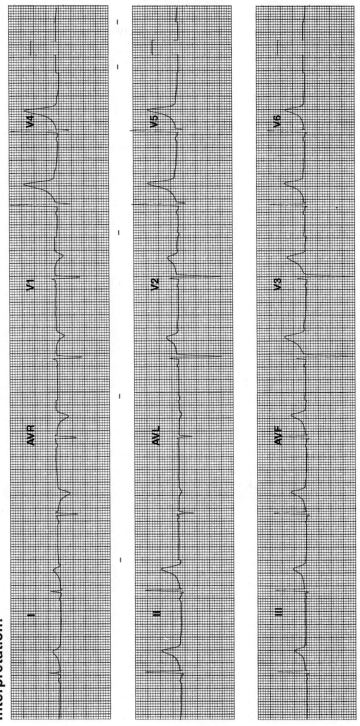

PRACTICE ECG 9

PR:

QRS:

QRS Axis:

Rate:

Interpretation:

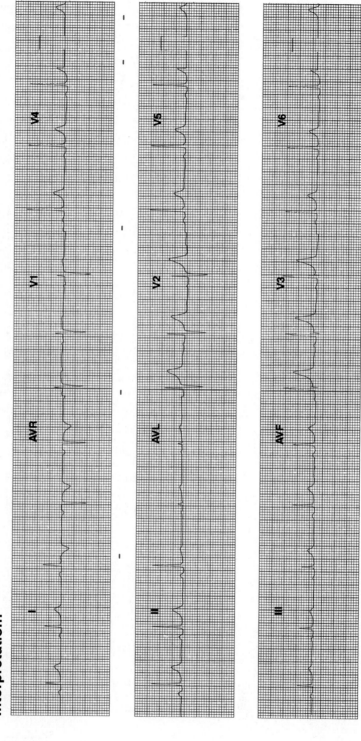

PRACTICE ECG 10

PR:

QRS:

QRS Axis:

Rate:

Interpretation:

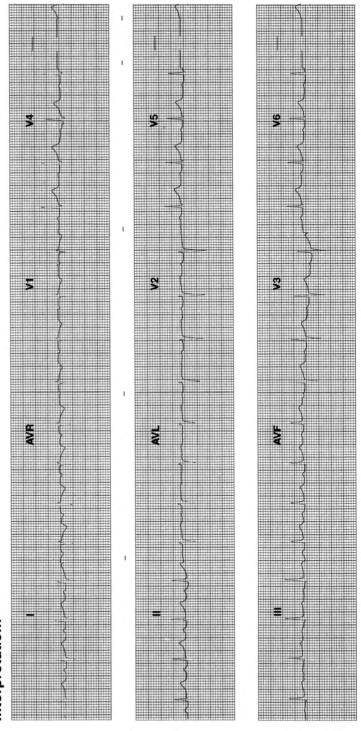

12-LEAD ECG INTERPRETATION

PRACTICE ECG 11

PR:

QRS:

QRS Axis:

Rate:

Interpretation:

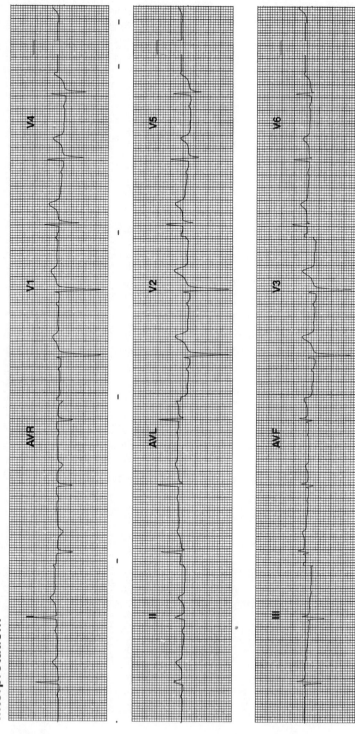

PRACTICE ECG 12

PR:

QRS:

QRS Axis:

Rate:

Interpretation:

12-LEAD ECG INTERPRETATION

PRACTICE ECG 13

PR:

QRS:

QRS Axis:

Rate:

Interpretation:

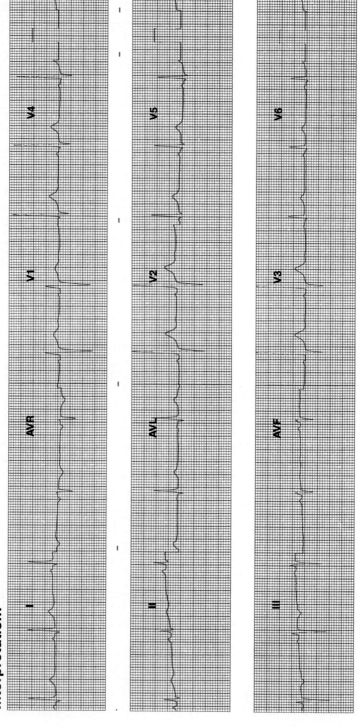

PRACTICE ECG 14

PR:

QRS:

QRS Axis:

Rate:

Interpretation:

PRACTICE ECG 15

PR:

QRS:

QRS Axis:

Rate:

Interpretation:

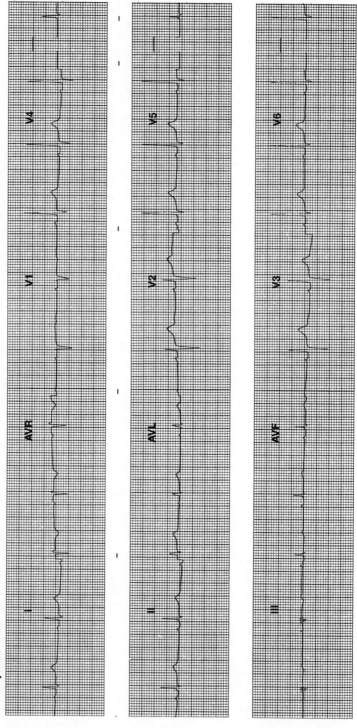

ANSWERS FOR PRACTICE ECGS

	PR	QRS	Axis	Rate	Interpretation
1.	.20	.06	+60°	96	Sinus rhythm
2.	.22	.06	+60°	97	Sinus rhythm with first degree AV block
3.	.16	.06	+60°	115	Sinus tachycardia
4.	.16	.08	−30°	60	Sinus rhythm with left axis
5.	.16	.08	+60°	101	Sinus tachycardia
6.	.18	.10	−30°	88	Sinus rhythm with left axis
7.	.10	.06	0°	78	Sinus rhythm with accelerated AV conduction
8.	.14	.08	+60°	50	Sinus bradycardia
9.	.18	.06	+60°	65	Sinus rhythm
10.	.20	.06	+90°	96	Sinus rhythm with right axis
11.	.22	.08	0°	59	Sinus bradycardia with first degree AV block
12.	.16	.08	+60°	51	Sinus bradycardia
13.	.14	.08	−30°	56	Sinus bradycardia with left axis
14.	.20	.08	+30°	73	Sinus rhythm
15.	.16	.08	+30°	57	Sinus bradycardia

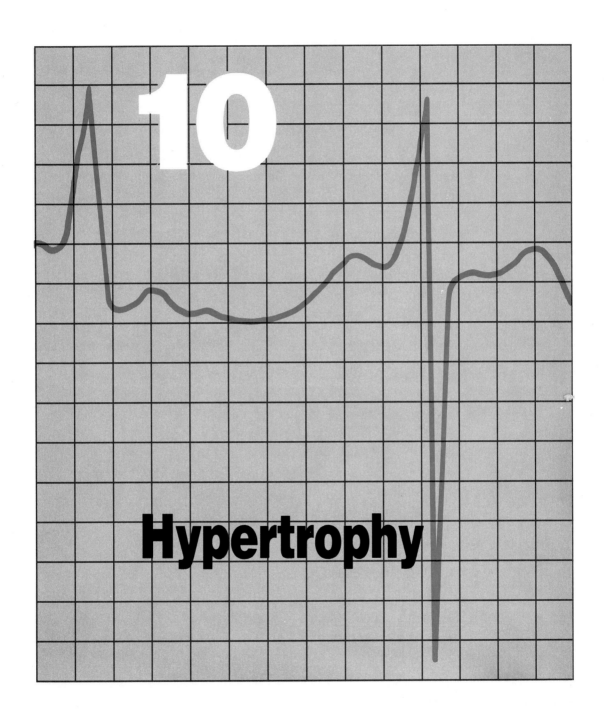

10

Hypertrophy

Hypertrophy is an increase in the thickness of the muscular wall of one of the chambers of the heart. Either or both of the atrial or ventricular walls can hypertrophy, and this is usually the result of a pressure or flow overload. Another term, often used interchangeably with hypertrophy, is *enlargement.*

ATRIAL

Left Atrial Hypertrophy. An increase in the size of the left atrial wall is called *left atrial hypertrophy*. The SA node initiates depolarization of the right atrium first, anteriorly and inferiorly toward the AV node, which we will label vector 1. Then the left atrium depolarizes in a posterior and leftward direction because it is located behind and to the left of the right atrium, and it is represented by vector 2.

NORMAL ATRIAL DEPOLARIZATION RECORDED IN V_1

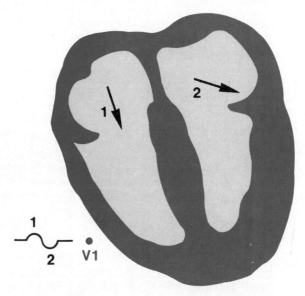

If we view atrial depolarization in lead V_1 on an ECG we will usually see a diaphasic P wave. The initial vector in the atria representing right atrial depolarization will be traveling toward V_1, and will inscribe an initial positive component of the P wave. The left atrial vector will be moving away from the V_1 electrode and will record a negative terminal portion of the P wave. If the left atrial wall is hypertrophied, there will be an increase in the amount of vectors traveling toward the left atrium, away from the V₁ electrode. This will cause the terminal portion of the P wave in V_1, representing left atrial depolarization, to enlarge to 1 mm or more deep.

ATRIAL DEPOLARIZATION

1. **Right atrial depolarization moving toward V_1 inscribes an initial positive deflection of the P wave.**
2. **Left atrial depolarization moving away from V_1 records a terminal negative deflection of the P wave.**

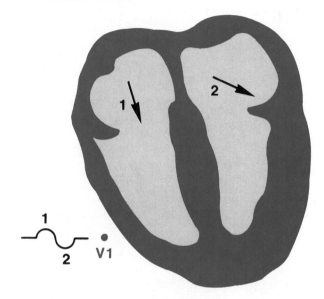

Normal Heart

1. **Right atrial depolarization moving toward V_1 inscribes an initial positive deflection of the P wave.**
2. **Depolarization of the enlarged left atrium moving away from V_1 produces a deeply inverted terminal portion of the P wave.**

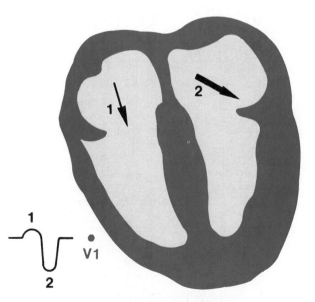

Left Atrial Hypertrophy

V₁ P WAVE CONFIGURATIONS

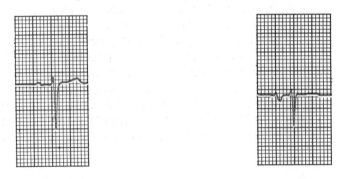

Normal   **Left Atrial Hypertrophy**

LEFT ATRIAL HYPERTROPHY

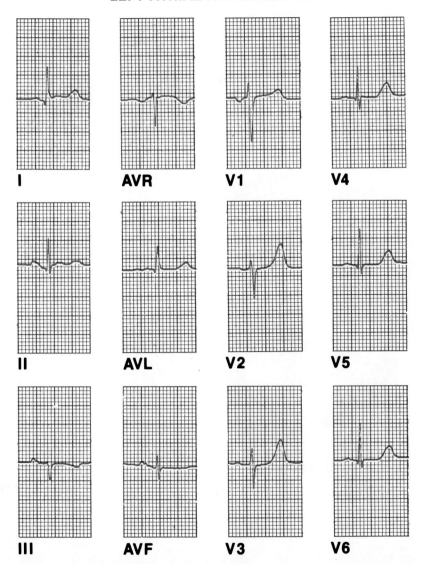

I	AVR	V1	V4
II	AVL	V2	V5
III	AVF	V3	V6

Right Atrial Hypertrophy. An increase in the size of the right atrial wall is called *right atrial hypertrophy*. If we use lead II to view atrial depolarization in a normal heart, we will notice an upright P wave not more than 2.4 mm high. The initial portion of atrial depolarization is represented by vector 1, which is traveling anteriorly and inferiorly toward lead II in a direct path, and which inscribes an upright deflection of the P wave. The second component of atrial depolarization is represented by vector 2, which is moving leftward and posteriorly, and only in the general direction of lead II; therefore it records a positive deflection of the P wave but with less voltage than vector 1.

NORMAL ATRIAL DEPOLARIZATION RECORDED IN LEAD II

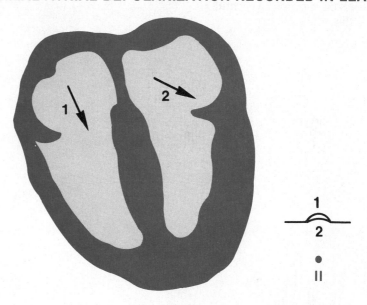

If the right atrium is hypertrophied, there will be an increase in the amount of vectors traveling directly toward lead II, and a P wave higher than 2.4 mm will be recorded.

ATRIAL DEPOLARIZATION

1. Depolarization of the right atrium traveling toward II inscribes a positive deflection of the P wave.
2. Depolarization of the left atrium moving toward II records a positive deflection of the P wave.

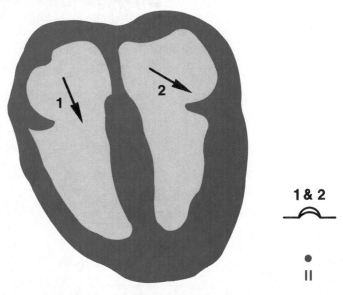

Normal Heart

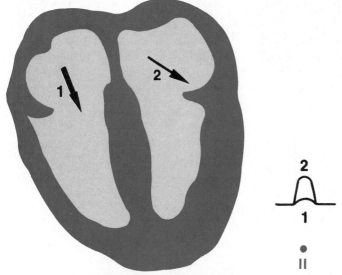

1. Depolarization of the enlarged right atrium moving toward lead II inscribes a tall peaked P wave.
2. Depolarization of the left atrium moving toward lead II records a small upright P almost simultaneously with the right atrium.

Right Atrial Hypertrophy

HOW TO QUICKLY AND ACCURATELY MASTER ECG INTERPRETATION

LEAD II P WAVE CONFIGURATIONS

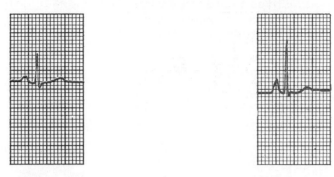

Normal   Right Atrial Hypertrophy

RIGHT ATRIAL HYPERTROPHY

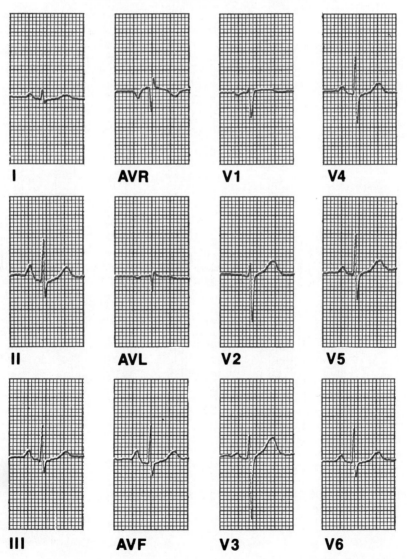

I   AVR   V1   V4

II   AVL   V2   V5

III   AVF   V3   V6

Biatrial Hypertrophy. An enlargement of both the left and the right atria is called *biatrial hypertrophy*. The criteria for recognition are those of left and right atrial hypertrophy.

BIATRIAL HYPERTROPHY

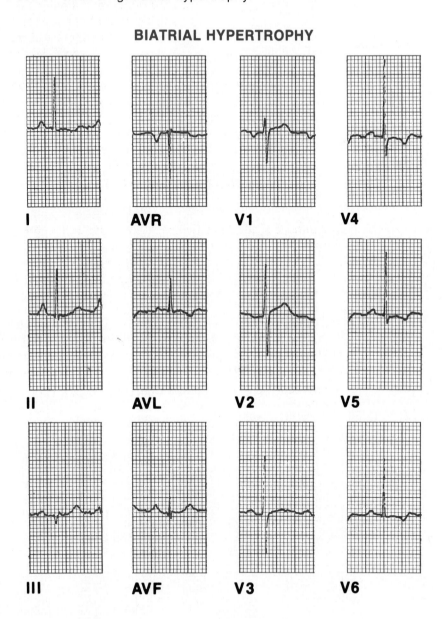

VENTRICULAR

The first stage of ventricular depolarization in the normal heart depicts septal activation and early right ventricular depolarization. V_1 will demonstrate a small R wave as depolarization travels toward it, and V_6 will show an initial small Q wave as depolarization proceeds away from it. The second stage of ventricular depolarization denotes apical activation. V_1 receives a negative deflection in the form of an S wave as depolarization moves away from it, and V_6 inscribes an R wave as depolarization is traveling toward it. In the last stage of ventricular depolarization, V_1 receives an increase in the size of the S wave while the main forces of depolarization, representing predominantly left ventricular depolarization, are moving away from it, and V_6 increases the R wave voltage as the wave of depolarization is moving toward it.

Left Ventricular Hypertrophy. An increase in the size of the wall of the left ventricle is called *left ventricular hypertrophy*. The left ventricular wall is approximately three times as thick as the right in a normal heart. When the wall of the left ventricle increases in thickness even more, large voltages are recorded in the leads over the hypertrophied left ventricle. Leads I, aVL, V_5, and V_6 will record the largest voltages in the form of tall R waves as the wave of depolarization moves toward them, and the right ventricular leads, V_1 and V_2, will increase their negative voltages as the wave of depolarization moves away from them. The increase in the muscle thickness of the ventricular walls increases the voltages over the hypertrophied area.

VENTRICULAR DEPOLARIZATION

The left ventricular wall is thicker than the right, causing the mean QRS vector to point leftward, rendering a large R wave in V_6 as the mean wave of depolarization moves toward the electrode, and recording a large S wave in V_1 as the mean wave of depolarization moves away from the electrode.

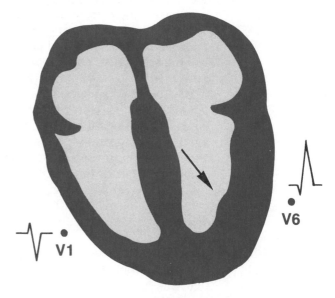

Normal Heart

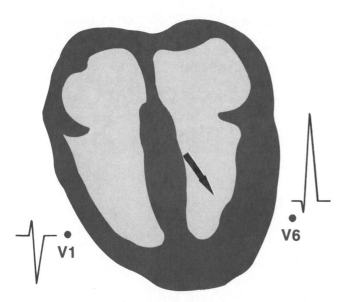

Left Ventricular Hypertrophy

The left ventricular wall increases in thickness, increasing the positive voltages in the leads over the hypertrophied area and increasing the negative voltages in the leads opposite the hypertrophied area.

A large R wave is recorded in V_6 as the mean wave of depolarization moves toward the electrode, and a large S wave is inscribed in V_1 as the mean wave of depolarization moves away from it.

Voltage criteria are used almost exclusively for the diagnosis of left ventricular hypertrophy on an ECG. We know that we will have large negative voltages in V_1 and large positive voltages in I, aVL, V_5, and V_6. The standard for recognition of left ventricular hypertrophy is:

S wave in V_1 + R wave in $V_5 \geq 35$ mm
   or
R wave in aVL ≥ 11 mm
   or
R wave in V_5 or $V_6 > 27$ mm

Repolarization changes, in the form of ST depression and asymmetrical T wave inversion, are often present in the left heart leads, although the reasons for these changes are not entirely clear.

REPOLARIZATION CHANGES WITH LEFT VENTRICULAR HYPERTROPHY

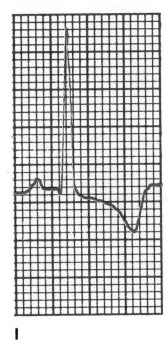

I

LVH & assoc. repolarization Δ's

Left axis deviation may also be present because of the increased voltages over the left side of the heart.

LEFT VENTRICULAR HYPERTROPHY

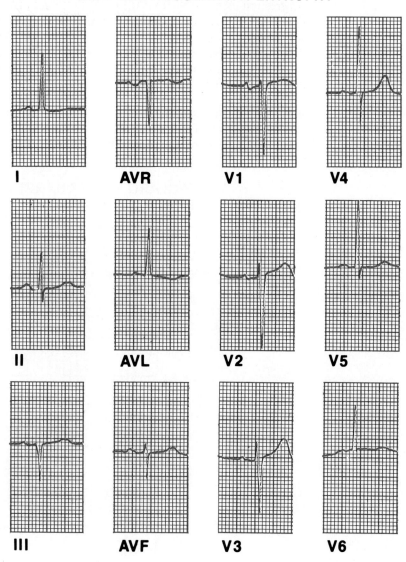

Right Ventricular Hypertrophy. An increase in the size of the walls of the right ventricle is called *right ventricular hypertrophy*. When the wall of the right ventricle increases in thickness, it can equal or exceed the thickness of the left ventricle. If it does not suprass the left ventricular thickness, then right ventricular hypertrophy may go unnoticed on an ECG. If the hypertrophy becomes severe, leads V_1 and V_2 will increase their R wave voltages, as the initial wave of depolarization moves toward the hypertrophied ventricle. The increase in the muscle thickness of the right ventricular wall increases the voltages in the leads over the hypertrophied area.

VENTRICULAR DEPOLARIZATION

The left ventricular wall is thicker than the right causing the mean QRS vector to point leftward, rendering a large R wave in V_6 as the mean wave of depolarization moves toward the electrode, and recording a large S wave in V_1 as the mean wave of depolarization moves away from the electrode.

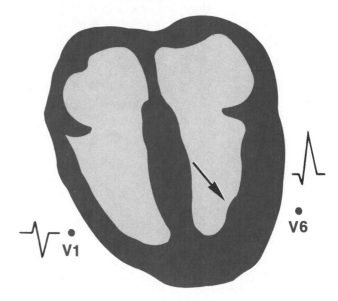

Normal Heart

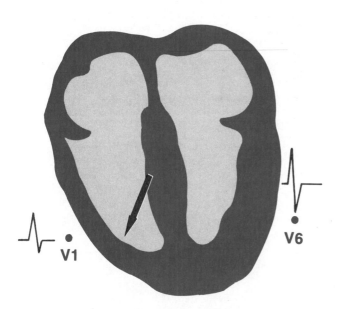

Right Ventricular Hypertrophy

The right ventricular wall increases in thickness, increasing the positive voltages in the leads over the hypertrophied area and increasing the negative voltages in the leads opposite the hypertrophied area.

A large R wave is recorded in V_1 as the mean wave of depolarization moves toward the electrode and a large S wave is inscribed in V_6 as the mean wave of depolarization moves away from it.

Voltage is one of the two criteria used for recognition of right ventricular hypertrophy:

R wave $\geq$ S wave in V_1
  or
R wave in V_1 + S wave in $V_6 \geq 11$ mm

Repolarization changes are often present in the right heart leads in the forms of ST depression and asymmetrical T wave inversion.

REPOLARIZATION CHANGES WITH RIGHT VENTRICULAR HYPERTROPHY

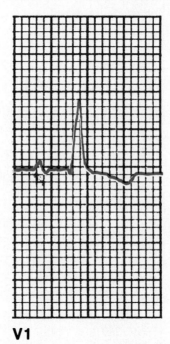

V1

The second criterion necessary for right ventricular hypertrophy is right axis deviation of +90° or greater. The axis shifts to the right in response to the greater amount of vectors present over the right ventricle.

RIGHT VENTRICULAR HYPERTROPHY

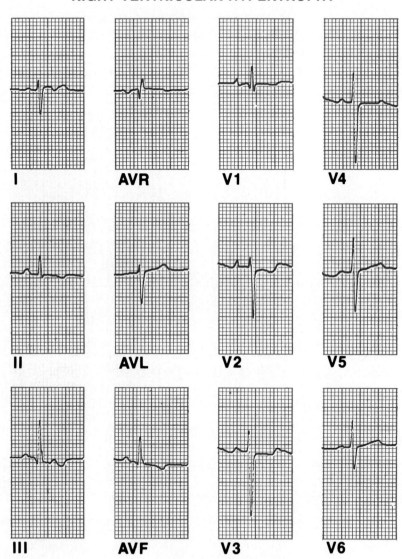

I AVR V1 V4

II AVL V2 V5

III AVF V3 V6

Biventricular Hypertrophy. An increase in the size of both the left and right ventricular walls is called *biventricular hypertrophy*. An enlargement of both ventricles may manifest voltage criteria for left ventricular hypertrophy with a QRS axis of +90° or greater, demonstrated by large voltages in leads II, III, and aVF, although ECG recognition of this abnormality is extremely difficult because biventricular hypertrophy tends to normalize a tracing.

BIVENTRICULAR HYPERTROPHY

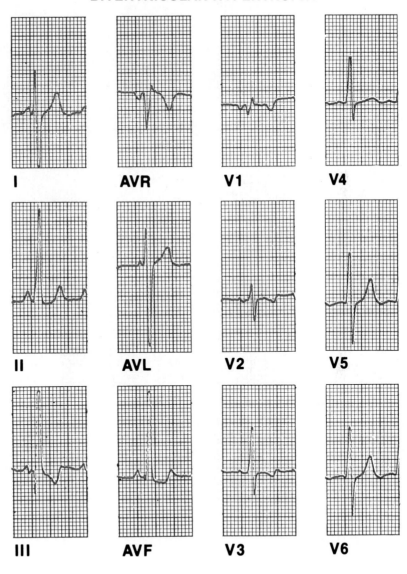

LEFT ATRIAL HYPERTROPHY

ECG Leads to Check for Left Atrial Hypertrophy

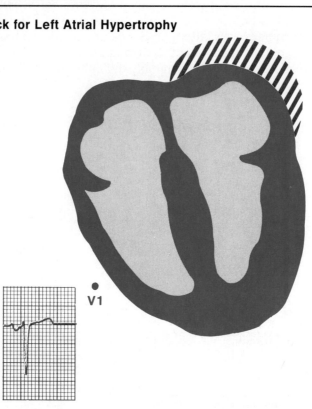

Criterion

Terminal portion of P wave in $V_1 \geq -1$ mm

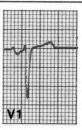

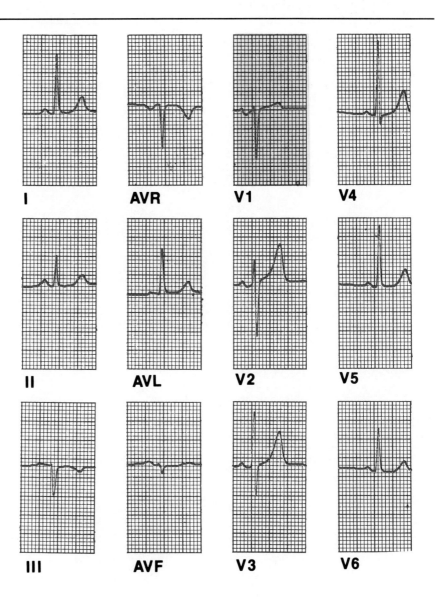

I   AVR   V1   V4

II   AVL   V2   V5

III   AVF   V3   V6

RIGHT ATRIAL HYPERTROPHY

ECG Leads to Check for Right Atrial Hypertrophy

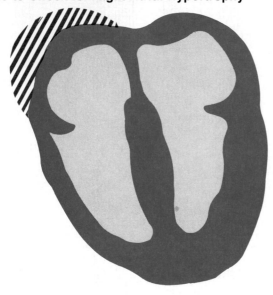

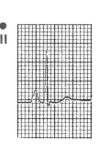

Criterion

Tall peaked P wave ≥ 2.5 mm in lead II

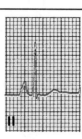

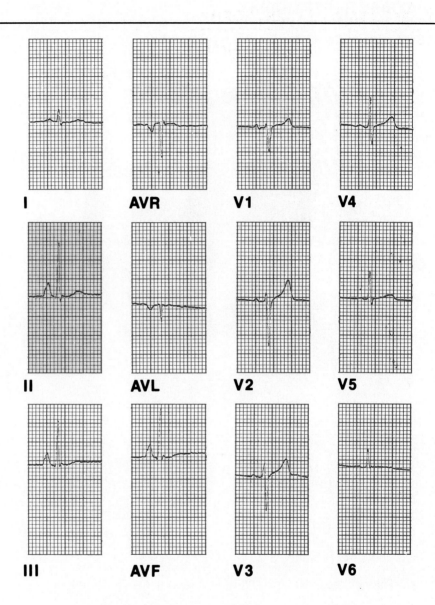

I   AVR   V1   V4

II   AVL   V2   V5

III   AVF   V3   V6

BIATRIAL HYPERTROPHY

ECG Leads to Check for Biatrial Hypertrophy

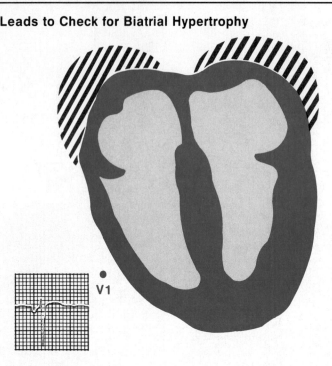

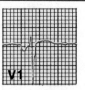

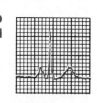

Criteria

1. Terminal portion of P wave in $V_1 \geq -1$ mm

2. Tall peaked P wave ≥ 2.5 mm in lead II

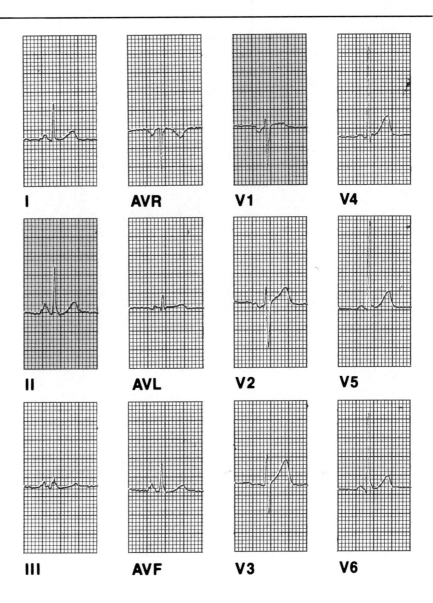

I   AVR   V1   V4

II   AVL   V2   V5

III   AVF   V3   V6

LEFT VENTRICULAR HYPERTROPHY

ECG Leads to Check for Left Ventricular Hypertrophy

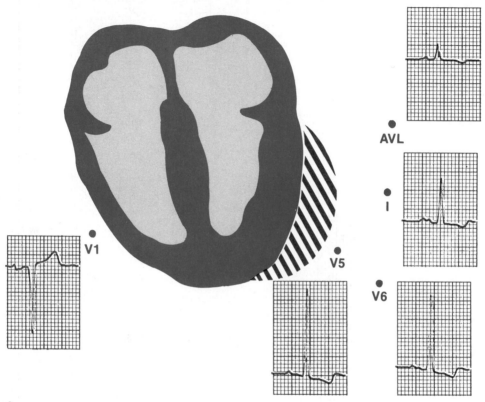

Criteria

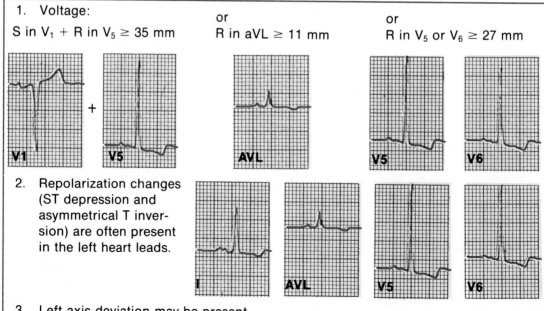

1. Voltage:
   S in V_1 + R in $V_5 \geq 35$ mm   or   R in aVL ≥ 11 mm   or   R in V_5 or $V_6 \geq 27$ mm

2. Repolarization changes (ST depression and asymmetrical T inversion) are often present in the left heart leads.

3. Left axis deviation may be present.

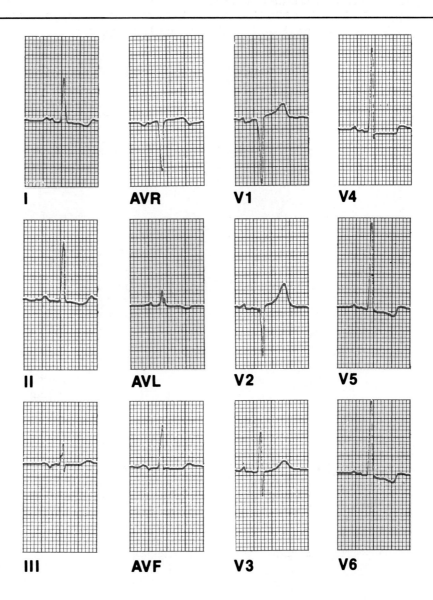

I AVR V1 V4

II AVL V2 V5

III AVF V3 V6

RIGHT VENTRICULAR HYPERTROPHY

ECG Leads to Check for Right Ventricular Hypertrophy

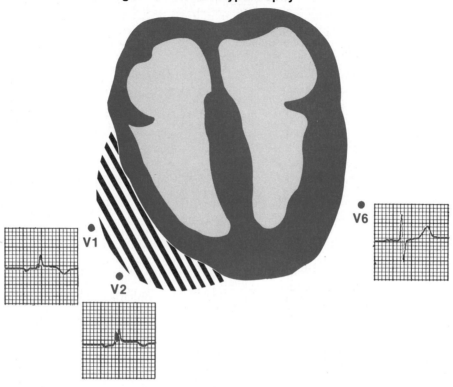

Criteria

1. Voltage:
   R wave $\geq$ S in V_1 or   R in V_1 + S in $V_6 \geq$ 11 mm

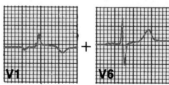

2. Right axis deviation of $+90°$ or greater

3. Repolarization changes (ST depression and asymmetrical T inversion) are often present in the right heart leads.

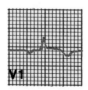 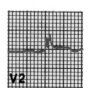

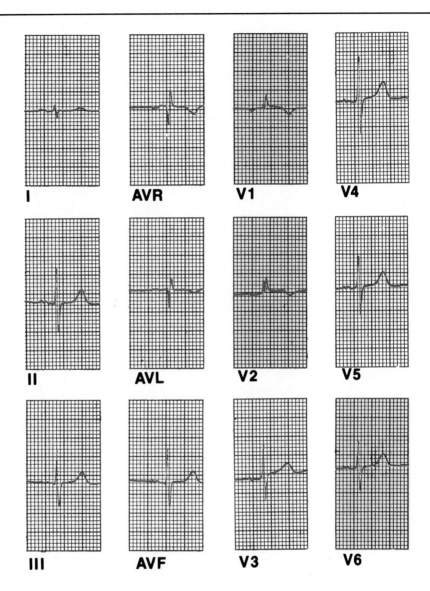

I AVR V1 V4

II AVL V2 V5

III AVF V3 V6

REVIEW ECG 1

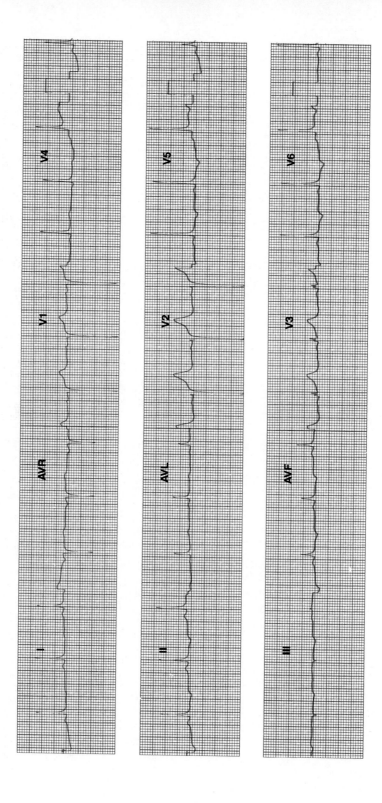

REVIEW ECG 2

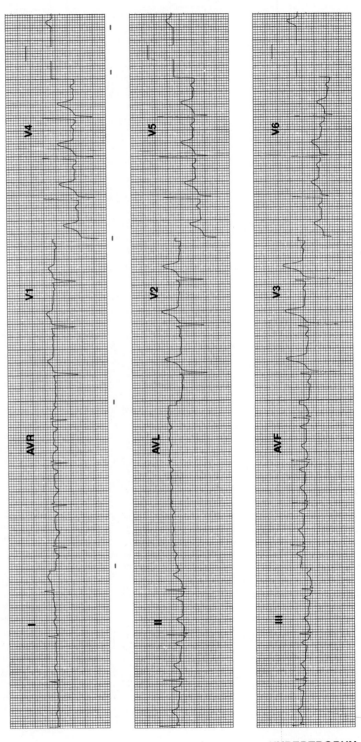

HYPERTROPHY

REVIEW ECG 3

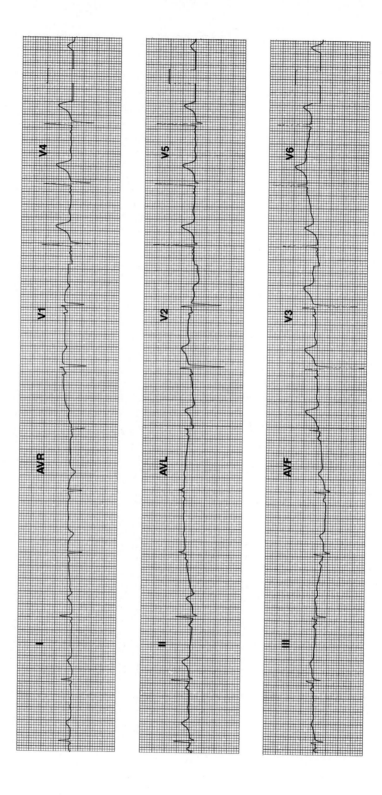

REVIEW ECG 4

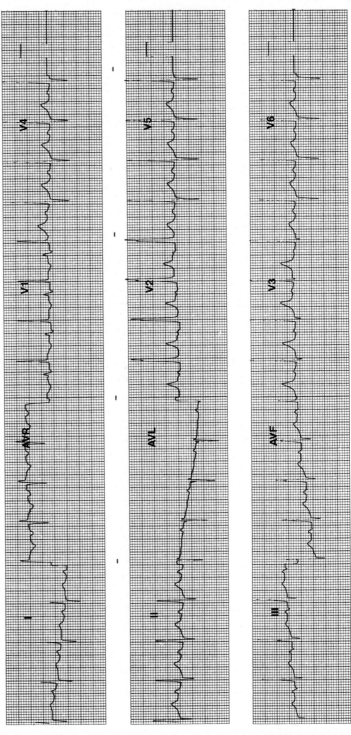

HYPERTROPHY

143

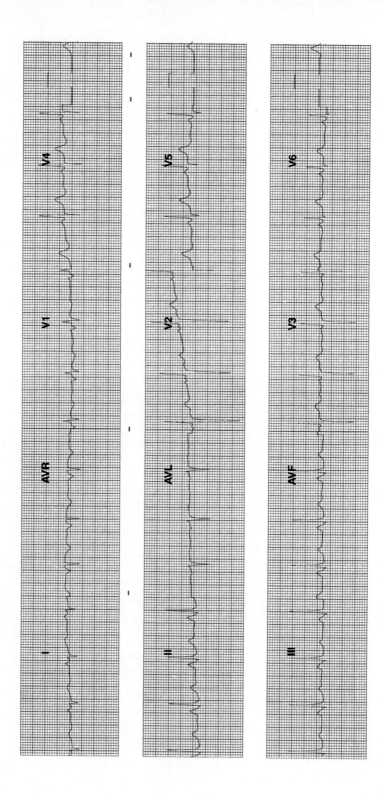

REVIEW ECG 6

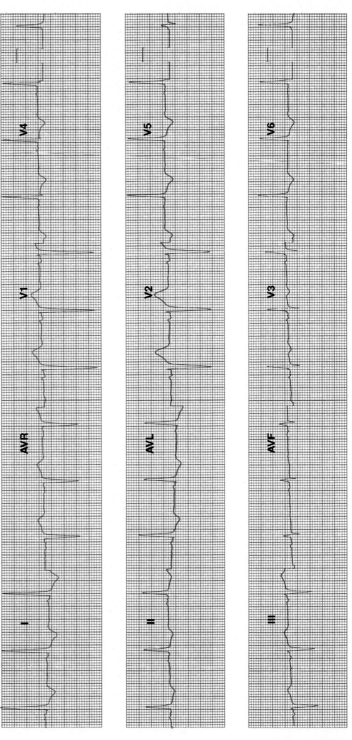

HYPERTROPHY

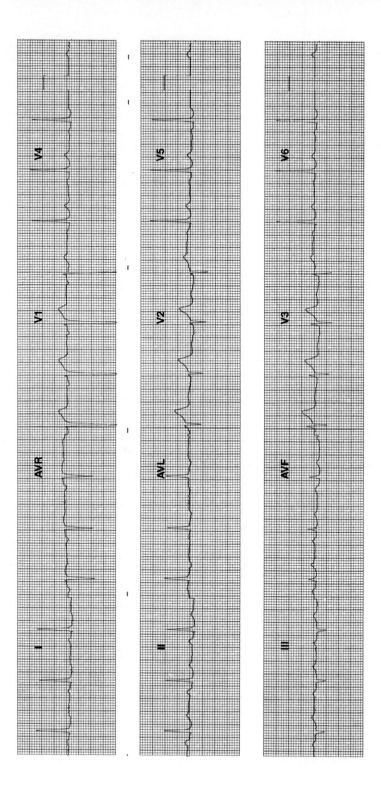

REVIEW ECG 8

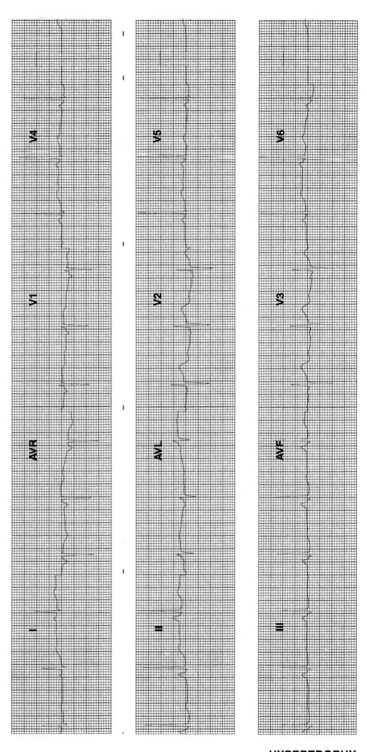

I   AVR   V1   V4

II   AVL   V2   V5

III   AVF   V3   V6

HYPERTROPHY

REVIEW ECG 9

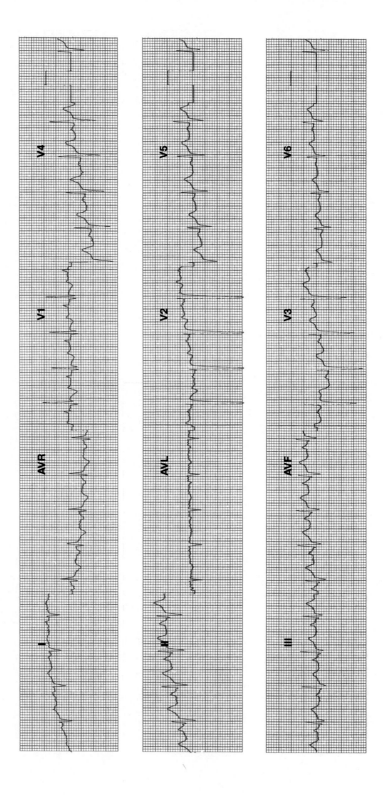

REVIEW ECG 10

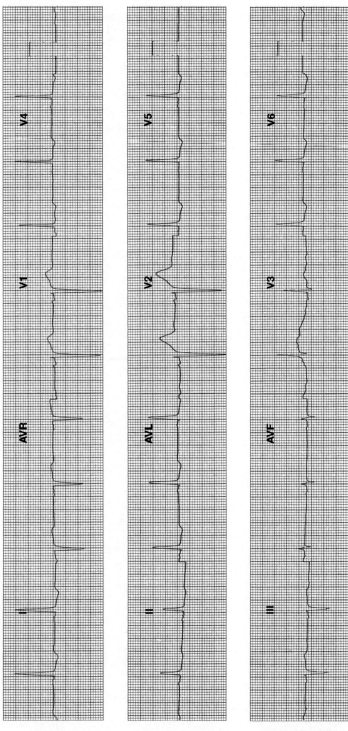

HYPERTROPHY

REVIEW ECG ANSWERS

1. Sinus rhythm at 72 per minute with left ventricular hypertrophy
2. Sinus rhythm at 89 per minute with right atrial enlargement
3. Sinus rhythm at 62 per minute with left atrial enlargement
4. Sinus rhythm at 96 per minute with left atrial enlargement
5. Sinus rhythm at 79 per minute with biatrial enlargement and right ventricular hypertrophy
6. Sinus rhythm at 68 per minute with left ventricular hypertrophy
7. Sinus rhythm at 76 per minute with left ventricular hypertrophy
8. Sinus rhythm at 68 per minute with biatrial enlargement
9. Sinus tachycardia at 109 per minute with right atrial enlargement and right ventricular hypertrophy
10. Sinus rhythm at 60 per minute with left ventricular hypertrophy

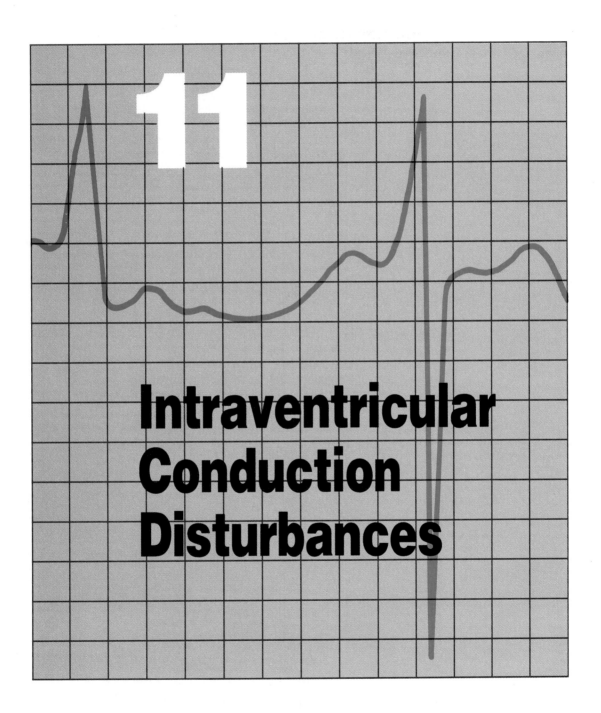

11

Intraventricular
Conduction
Disturbances

An intraventricular conduction disturbance is an abnormal conduction of an electrical impulse in one or more of the conduction pathways below the bundle of His: (1) right bundle branch, (2) left bundle branch, (3) left anterior fascicle, or (4) left posterior fascicle.

BUNDLE BRANCH BLOCK

Right Bundle Branch Block. A delay or blockage of conduction in the right bundle branch is called *right bundle branch block*. A normal cardiac impulse is initiated in the sinus node, travels through and depolarizes the atria, and transverses the AV node and bundle of His. The cardiac impulse then proceeds down the left bundle, initiates septal activation, and attempts to move down the right bundle at the same time. On finding the right bundle branch blocked, the electrical impulse advances through the left bundle into the anterior and posterior fascicles and into the Purkinje fibers of the left ventricle. The electrical impulse will then travel from the left ventricle across the septum, into the right ventricle, and will initiate depolarization.

The initial activation in the ventricles during right bundle branch block remains the same as that of the normal heart, since the septum depolarizes from left to right via the left bundle branch system. Lead V_1 will have an initial R wave inscribed, and lead I will have a Q wave recorded. The left ventricle depolarizes first, unopposed by the right, and inscribes an S wave while the forces of depolarization are moving away from the V_1 electrode, and lead I records an R wave as the wave of depolarization moves toward it. Finally, the right ventricle depolarizes, unopposed by the left. As the wave of depolarization moves toward the V_1 electrode an R' wave is inscribed, and as the wave of depolarization moves away from lead I, an S wave is displayed.

VENTRICULAR DEPOLARIZATION

The initial activation in the ventricles is rightward and in the direction of V_1, resulting in a small R wave in V_1 as the wave of depolarization moves toward it, and a small Q in V_6 as the wave of depolarization moves away from the electrode. Left and right ventricular depolarization occur almost simultaneously, demonstrating a mean QRS vector directed leftward and inferiorly toward V_6, inscribing a large R wave, and away from V_1, displaying a deep S wave in that lead.

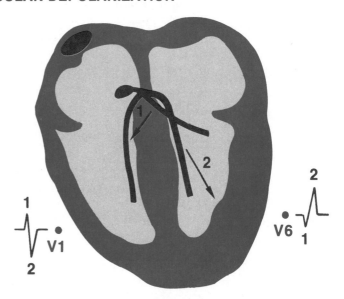

Normal Heart

Initial ventricular depolarization is normal, resulting in a small R in V_1 and a small Q in V_6. Because of the blockage in the right bundle branch, the left ventricle depolarizes first, recording an S wave in V_1 as the wave of depolarization moves away from the electrode and an R wave in V_6 as the wave of depolarization moves toward it. The right ventricle is then depolarized abnormally across the interventricular septum, recording an R' in V_1 as the wave of depolarization again travels toward that electrode, and an S wave in V_6 as the wave of depolarization travels away from it. Because of delay in conduction in the right ventricle, the terminal portion of the QRS is widened, resulting in a QRS of .12 second or greater.

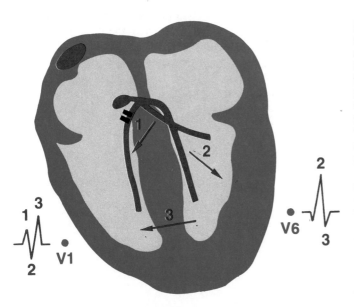

Right Bundle Branch Block

$QRS > .12s$

INTRAVENTRICULAR CONDUCTION DISTURBANCES

The characteristic findings of right bundle branch block are a QRS that is .12 second or greater in duration, a predominantly positive QRS in V_1, a wide S wave in lead I, and ST depression and T wave inversion, representing repolarization changes occurring with right bundle branch block. In the presence of right bundle branch block, right ventricular hypertrophy should not be diagnosed.

QRS CONFIGURATIONS

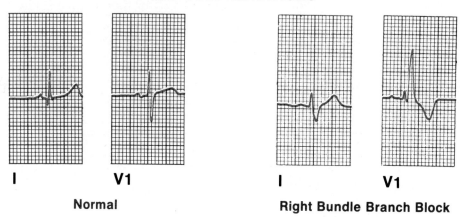

I	V1	I	V1
Normal		**Right Bundle Branch Block**	

RIGHT BUNDLE BRANCH BLOCK

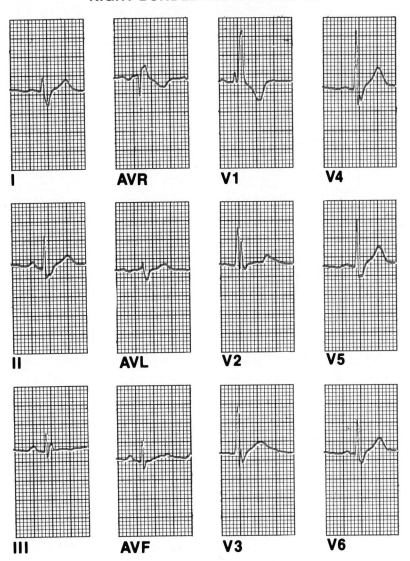

I AVR V1 V4

II AVL V2 V5

III AVF V3 V6

INTRAVENTRICULAR CONDUCTION DISTURBANCES

Left Bundle Branch Block. Delay or blockage of conduction in the main left bundle branch is called *left bundle branch block*. A cardiac impulse begins in the sinus node and depolarizes the atria, travels through the AV node and the bundle of His, and arrives at the left and right bundle branches. The impulse proceeds down the right bundle branch and attempts to move down the left bundle branch. On finding the left side blocked, the wave of depolarization travels down the right bundle and initiates depolarization through the Purkinje fibers and travels across the septum to depolarize the left ventricle.

The initial activation in the ventricles during left bundle branch block is greatly changed from that of the normal heart. The septum is unable to be depolarized from left to right and is depolarized from right to left by way of the right bundle branch. Normal septal Q waves will not be seen in leads I, aVL, V_5, and V_6. Lead V_1 may show a small Q wave as the initial wave of depolarization moves away from it. The right ventricle depolarizes first, sometimes inscribing a small R wave in V_1 as the wave of depolarization moves toward it. Often, the small Q wave or R wave in V_1 will be absent, leaving only a QS wave. Lastly, the left ventricle depolarizes, unopposed by the right, and a large S wave is inscribed in V_1 as the wave of depolarization moves away from the electrode.

loss of septal Q wave

VENTRICULAR DEPOLARIZATION

The initial activation in the ventricles is rightward and in the direction of V_1, resulting in a small R wave in V_1 as the wave of depolarization moves toward it, and a small Q in V_6 as the wave of depolarization moves away from the electrode. Left and right ventricular depolarization occur almost simultaneously, demonstrating a mean QRS vector directed leftward and inferiorly toward V_6, inscribing a large R wave, and away from V_1, displaying a deep S wave in that lead.

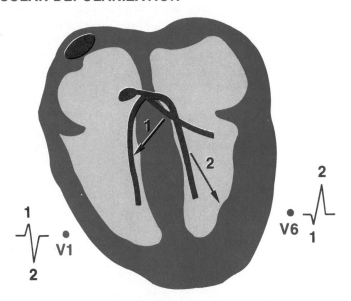

Normal Heart

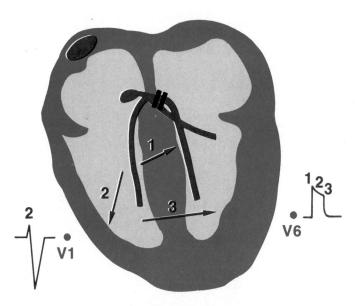

Left Bundle Branch Block

Because the left bundle branch is blocked, the septum depolarizes in a rightward direction, traveling toward V_6 and recording an R wave in it, and away from V_1, inscribing a tiny Q wave, which is often not visible. The right ventricle depolarizes first, inscribing a small R wave in V_1 as the wave of depolarization moves toward the electrode, and an S wave or slurred R wave in V_6 as the wave of depolarization moves away from it. The left ventricle is then depolarized abnormally through the interventricular septum, recording a deep S wave in V_1 as the wave of depolarization moves away from the electrode, and an R' in V_6 as the wave of depolarization moves toward it. Because of delay in conduction through the left ventricle, the entire QRS complex is widened to .12 second or greater.

INTRAVENTRICULAR CONDUCTION DISTURBANCES

The characteristic hallmarks of left bundle branch block are a widened and bizarre QRS complex that is .12 second or greater in duration, and a QRS that is predominantly negative in V_1. Septal Q waves will be absent in leads I, aVL, V_5, and V_6. ST depression and T wave inversion, representing repolarization changes of left bundle branch block, will be seen. Left ventricular hypertrophy should not be diagnosed in the presence of left bundle branch block.

V_1 QRS CONFIGURATIONS

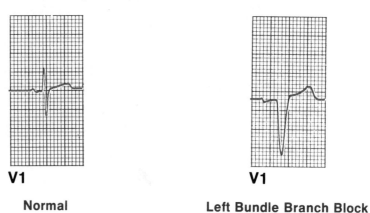

V1

Normal

V1

Left Bundle Branch Block

LEFT BUNDLE BRANCH BLOCK

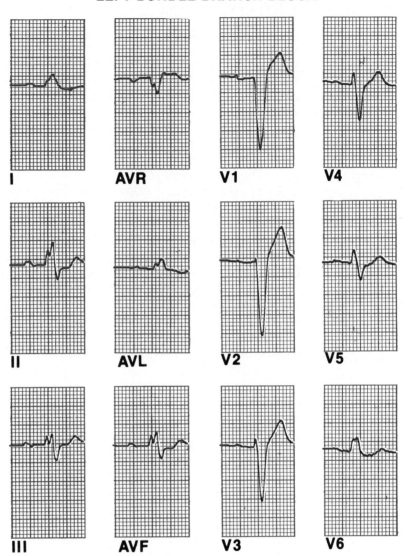

I	AVR	V1	V4
II	AVL	V2	V5
III	AVF	V3	V6

INTRAVENTRICULAR CONDUCTION DISTURBANCES

HEMIBLOCK

Left Anterior Hemiblock. Delay or blockage of the anterior fascicle of the left bundle branch is called *left anterior hemiblock.* The electrical impulse arrives at the bundle of His after depolarizing the atria and traveling through the AV node. The impulse then travels to the right and left bundle branches and is blocked at the anterior division of the left bundle. The depolarization wave travels down the posterior fascicle and through the connection of Purkinje fibers between the two fascicles, the anterior portion of the left ventricle is depolarized.

The initial activation in the ventricles remains the same as in a normal heart, since the septum depolarizes from left to right via the remaining fascicle. Lead I will have a Q wave recorded as the wave of depolarization moves away from the electrode, and lead III will display an initial R wave as the wave of depolarization moves toward it. The right bundle branch depolarizes normally, and the left bundle branch depolarizes in a slightly different way. The posterior fascicle depolarizes the posterior portion of the left ventricle, and then the anterior portion is depolarized with a minimum of delay through the connections of the Purkinje fibers with the posterior division. The main wave of depolarization will be oriented superiorly toward lead I rather than leftward and laterally. This will produce an R wave in lead I and an S wave in lead III.

VENTRICULAR DEPOLARIZATION

The initial activation in the ventricles is rightward and in the direction of III, resulting in a small R in III as the wave of depolarization moves toward it, and a small Q wave in I as the wave of depolarization travels away from the electrode. Left and right ventricular depolarization occur almost simultaneously, demonstrating a mean QRS vector directed leftward toward lead I, inscribing an R wave, and inferiorly toward lead III also displaying an R wave, or variable patterns of R and S waves.

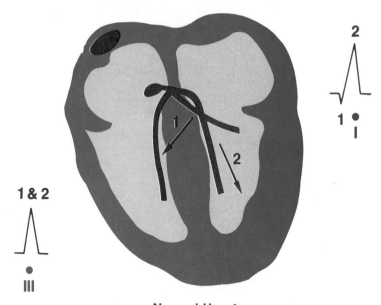

Normal Heart

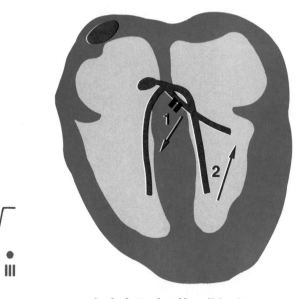

Left Anterior Hemiblock

The initial activation in the ventricles is usually rightward, traveling toward III and inscribing a small R wave, and away from I, recording a small Q wave. The mean QRS vector remains leftward but because of the blockage in the left anterior branch, the mean QRS vector now becomes superior, resulting in a deep S wave in III as the wave of depolarization moves away from the electrode, and an R wave in I as the wave of depolarization travels toward it.

INTRAVENTRICULAR CONDUCTION DISTURBANCES

The characteristic signs of left anterior hemiblock are an axis shift to −40° or greater, a small Q wave in lead I, and no evidence of inferior infarction (see Chapter 12). If left anterior hemiblock is present, the voltage criterion for left ventricular hypertrophy in aVL is increased to 16 mm or greater.

LEFT ANTERIOR HEMIBLOCK

I AVR V1 V4

II AVL V2 V5

III AVF V3 V6

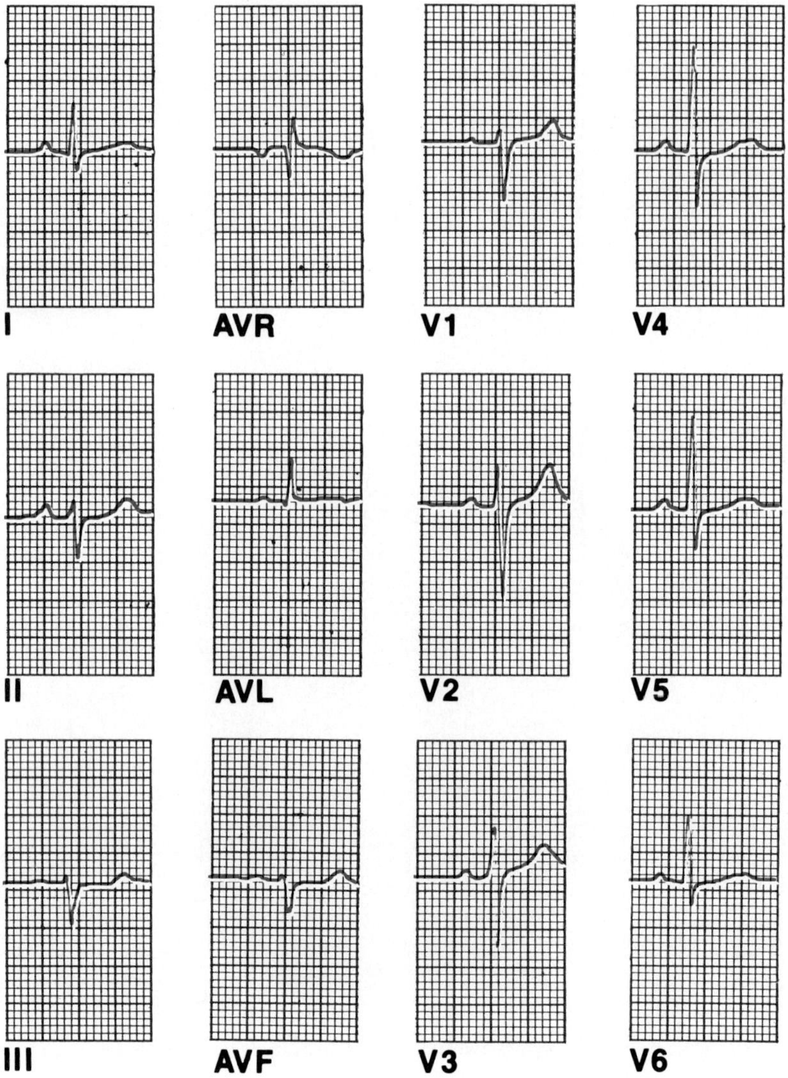

Left Posterior Hemiblock. Delay or blockage of the posterior fascicle of the left bundle branch is called *left posterior hemiblock*. The electrical impulse arrives at the right and left bundle branches after traveling through normal conduction pathways. Conduction proceeds down the right bundle branch normally. Conduction is either delayed or blocked at the posterior division of the left bundle branch, so the impulse travels down the anterior fascicle and through the connection of Purkinje fibers between the two fascicles; the posterior portion of the left ventricle is depolarized.

Although septal activation still occurs, the majority of the forces of initial depolarization in the ventricles are moving superiorly and leftward by way of the anterior fascicle toward lead I, recording an R wave, and are moving away from lead III, displaying a Q wave.

After the superior portion of the left ventricle is depolarized by way of the anterior fascicle, the inferior portion will be depolarized by the connections of Purkinje fibers between the two fascicles. The main wave of depolarization is projected inferiorly, toward lead III, recording an R wave, and away from lead I, producing an S wave.

VENTRICULAR DEPOLARIZATION

The initial activation in the ventricles is rightward and in the direction of III, resulting in a small R in III as the wave of depolarization moves toward it, and a small Q wave in I as the wave of depolarization travels away from the electrode. Left and right ventricular depolarization occur almost simultaneously, demonstrating a mean QRS vector directed leftward toward lead I, inscribing an R wave, and inferiorly toward lead III also displaying an R wave, or variable patterns of R and S waves.

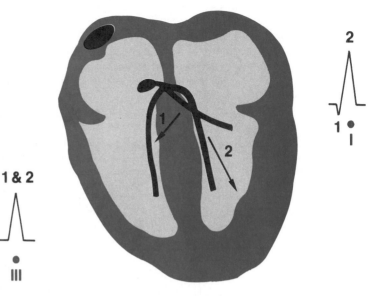

Normal Heart

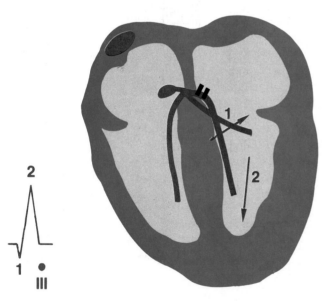

The initial activation in the ventricles is leftward, traveling toward I and recording a small R wave, and away from III, inscribing a Q wave. The mean QRS vector becomes rightward, and because of the blockage in the left posterior branch, the mean QRS vector now becomes inferior, resulting in a large R wave in III as the wave of depolarization moves toward it, and a deep S wave in I as the wave of depolarization travels away from the electrode.

Left Posterior Hemiblock

The criteria for recognition of left posterior hemiblock are an axis shift to +120° or greater, a small Q wave in lead III, and no evidence of right ventricular hypertrophy.

LEFT POSTERIOR HEMIBLOCK

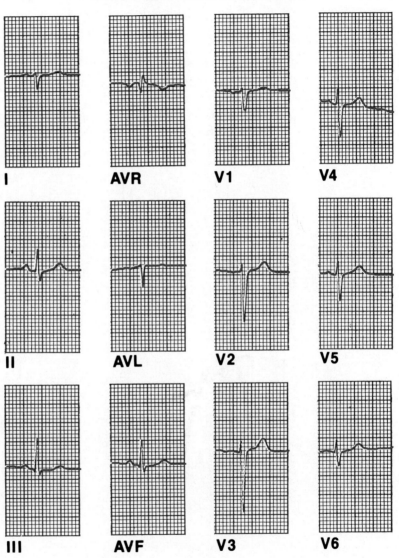

BIFASCICULAR BLOCK

Bifascicular block indicates blockage in more than one conducting fascicle in the ventricles:

1. Right bundle branch block and left anterior hemiblock
2. Right bundle branch block and left posterior hemiblock
3. Right or left bundle branch block with prolonged AV conduction in the remaining fascicle (first degree AV block—PR .20 second or greater)
4. Alternating right and left bundle branch block

1. Right bundle branch block and left anterior hemiblock are characterized by a QRS .12 second or greater, a wide S wave, and a small Q wave in lead I and a predominantly positive QRS in V_1, and a QRS axis of $-40°$ or greater.

RIGHT BUNDLE BRANCH BLOCK AND LEFT ANTERIOR HEMIBLOCK

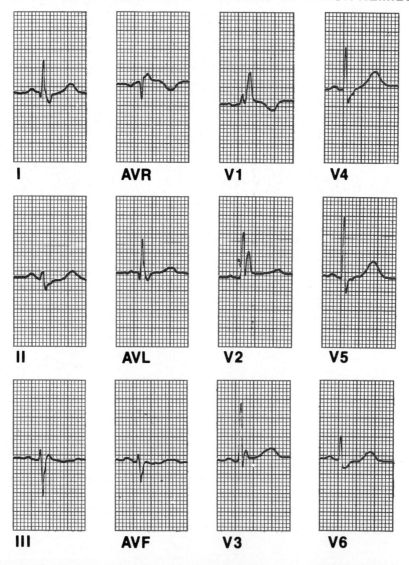

I	AVR	V1	V4
II	AVL	V2	V5
III	AVF	V3	V6

2. Right bundle branch block and left posterior hemiblock are recognized by a QRS .12 second or greater, a wide S wave in lead I, and a predominantly positive QRS in V₁, a QRS axis +120° or greater, and a small Q wave in lead III.

RIGHT BUNDLE BRANCH BLOCK AND LEFT POSTERIOR HEMIBLOCK

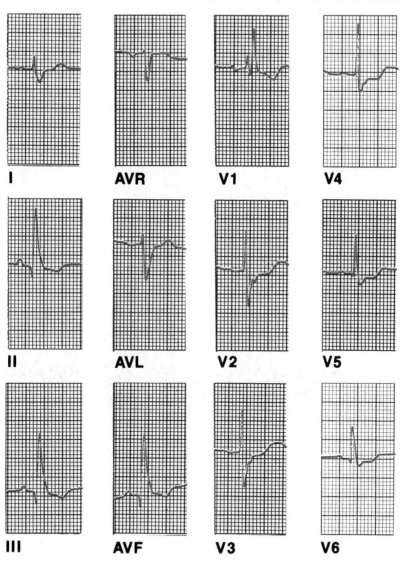

I	AVR	V1	V4
II	AVL	V2	V5
III	AVF	V3	V6

INTRAVENTRICULAR CONDUCTION DISTURBANCES

3. Right or left bundle branch block with first degree AV block is seen as right bundle branch block with a QRS .12 second or greater, a wide S wave in lead I, and a predominantly positive QRS in V_1 with a PR .20 second or greater; or it may be seen as left bundle branch block with a QRS .12 second or greater, a predominantly negative QRS in V_1, no evidence of septal Q waves in leads I, aVL, V_5 and V_6, and a PR .20 second or greater. If the first degree AV block represents delay in conduction in the AV node rather than in the remaining conducting fascicle, bifascicular block would not be present.

RIGHT BUNDLE BRANCH BLOCK AND FIRST DEGREE AV BLOCK

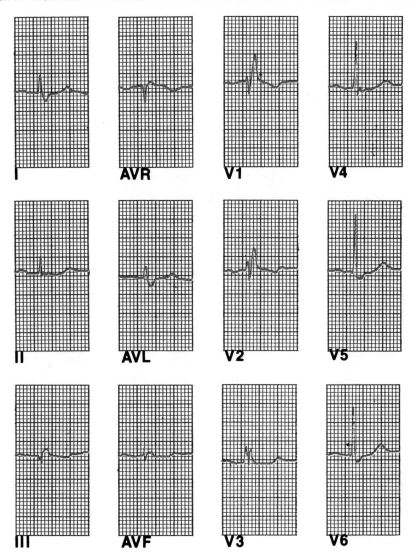

INTRAVENTRICULAR CONDUCTION DISTURBANCES

LEFT BUNDLE BRANCH BLOCK AND FIRST DEGREE AV BLOCK

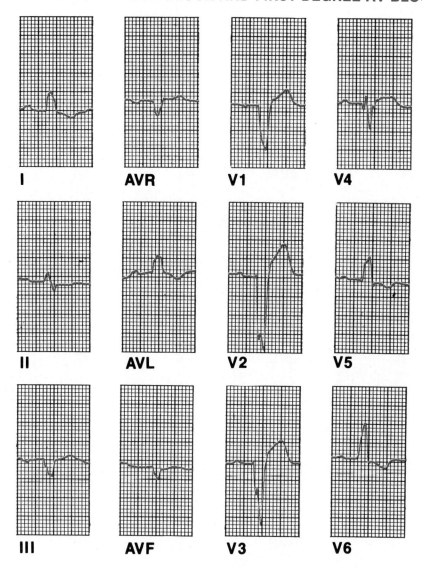

I   AVR   V1   V4

II   AVL   V2   V5

III   AVF   V3   V6

4. Alternating left and right bundle branch block is characterized by a left bundle branch block configuration, varying with a right bundle branch block pattern.

NONSPECIFIC INTRAVENTRICULAR CONDUCTION DISTURBANCE

A conduction abnormality located in the ventricles that is characterized by a QRS .12 second or greater that does not conform to either the left or right bundle branch block pattern is called *nonspecific intraventricular conduction disturbance.*

NONSPECIFIC INTRAVENTRICULAR CONDUCTION DISTURBANCE

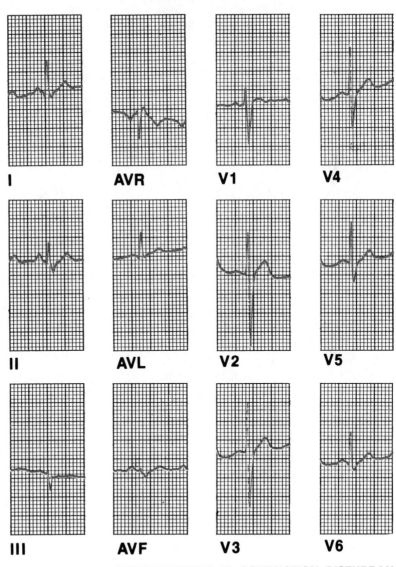

INTRAVENTRICULAR CONDUCTION DISTURBANCES

RIGHT BUNDLE BRANCH BLOCK

ECG Leads to Check for Right Bundle Branch Block

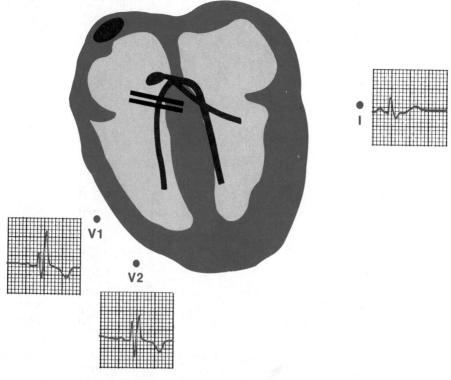

Criteria

1. QRS interval .12 second or greater

2. QRS predominantly positive in V_1

3. Wide S in lead I

4. Repolarization changes

5. Do not diagnose right ventricular hypertrophy in the presence of right bundle branch block.

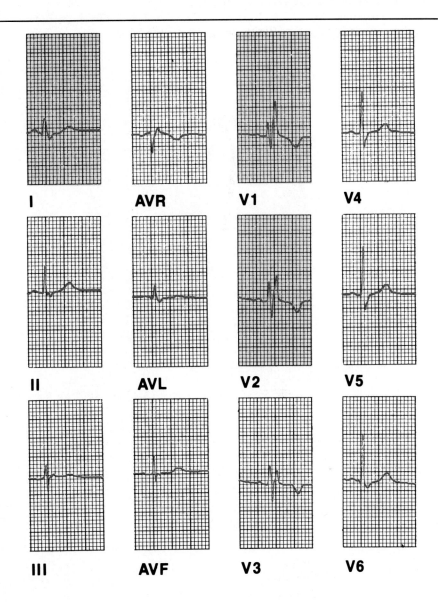

I   AVR   V1   V4

II   AVL   V2   V5

III   AVF   V3   V6

LEFT BUNDLE BRANCH BLOCK

ECG Leads to Check for Left Bundle Branch Block

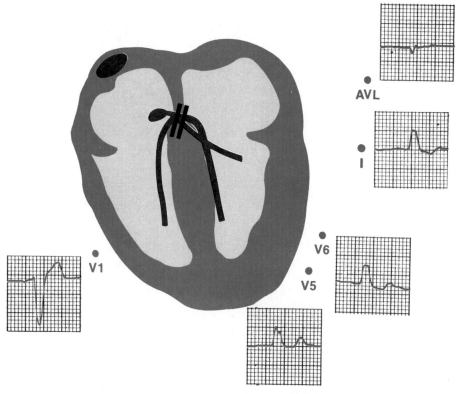

AVL

I

V1

V6

V5

Criteria

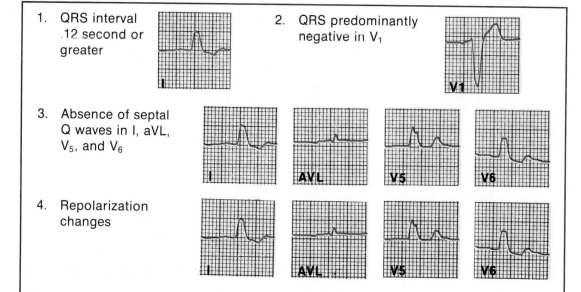

1. QRS interval .12 second or greater

   I

2. QRS predominantly negative in V_1

   V1

3. Absence of septal Q waves in I, aVL, V_5, and V_6

   I   AVL   V5   V6

4. Repolarization changes

   I   AVL   V5   V6

5. Do not diagnose left ventricular hypertrophy in the presence of left bundle branch block

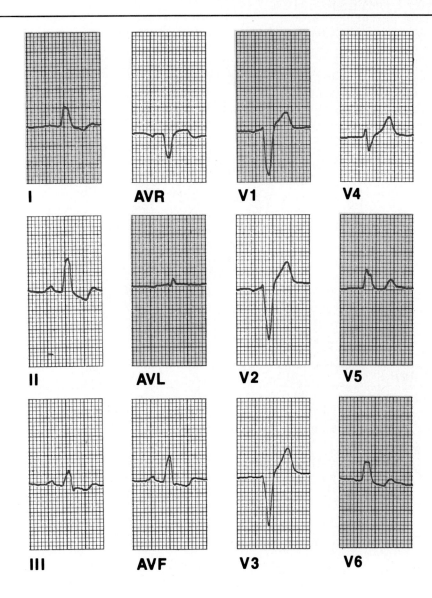

I	AVR	V1	V4
II	AVL	V2	V5
III	AVF	V3	V6

LEFT ANTERIOR HEMIBLOCK

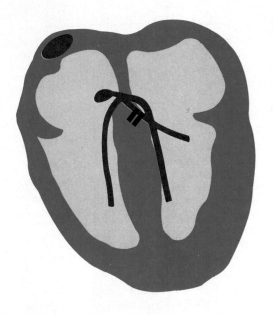

Criteria

1. Axis −40° or greater

2. No evidence of inferior infarction

3. Small Q wave in Lead I

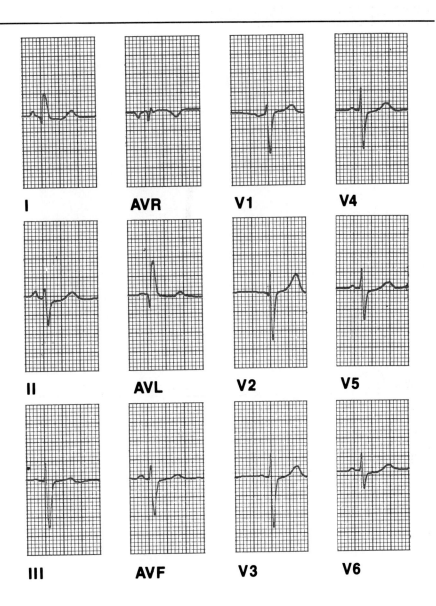

I AVR V1 V4

II AVL V2 V5

III AVF V3 V6

LEFT POSTERIOR HEMIBLOCK

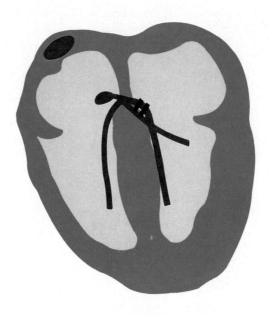

Criteria

1. Axis +120° or greater

2. No evidence of right ventricular hypertrophy

3. Small Q wave in Lead III

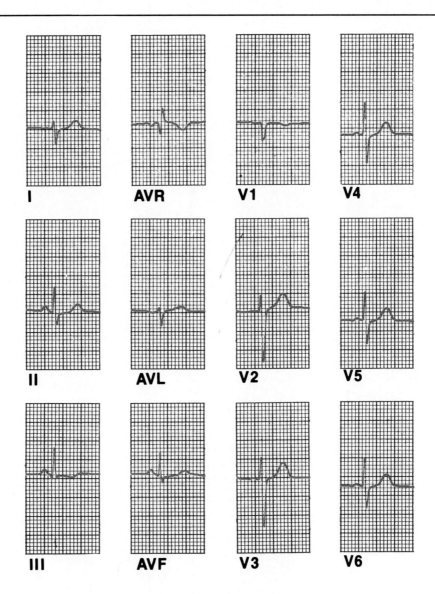

I AVR V1 V4

II AVL V2 V5

III AVF V3 V6

INTRAVENTRICULAR CONDUCTION DISTURBANCES

REVIEW ECG 1

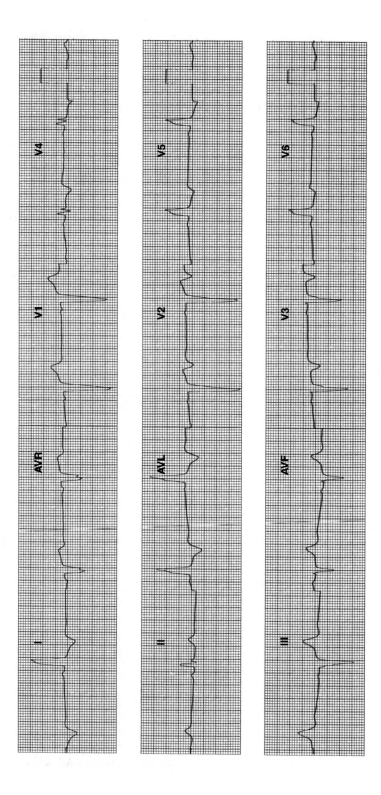

REVIEW ECG 2

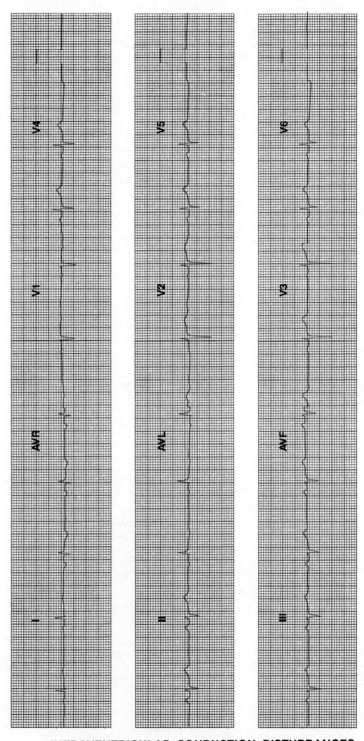

INTRAVENTRICULAR CONDUCTION DISTURBANCES

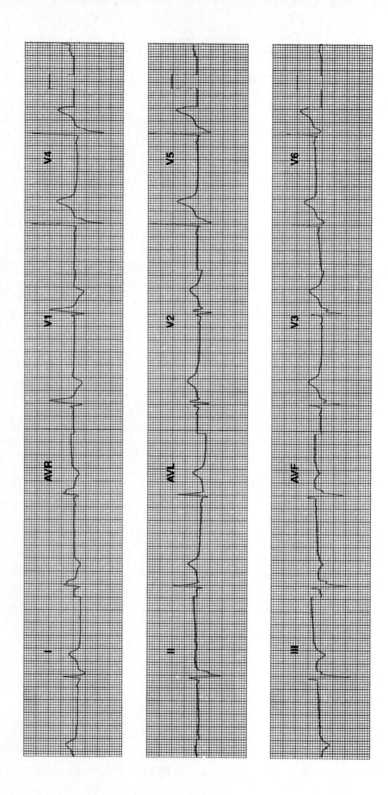

REVIEW ECG 4

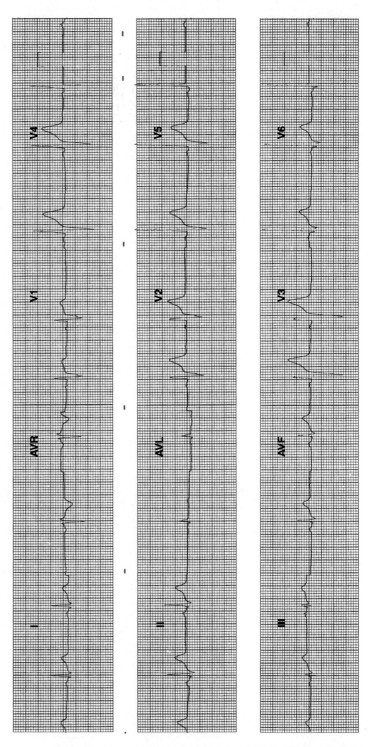

INTRAVENTRICULAR CONDUCTION DISTURBANCES

183

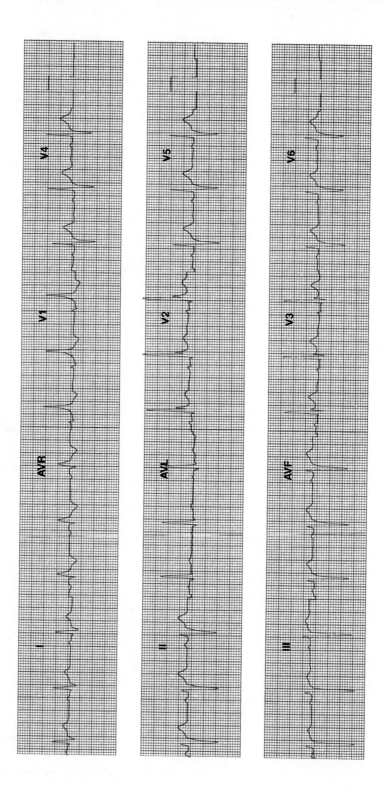

REVIEW ECG 6

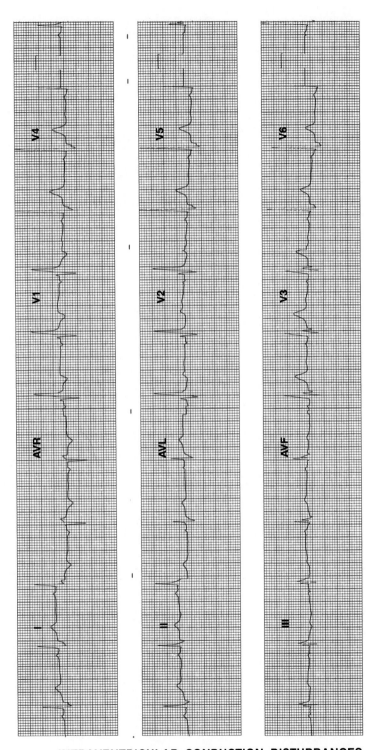

INTRAVENTRICULAR CONDUCTION DISTURBANCES

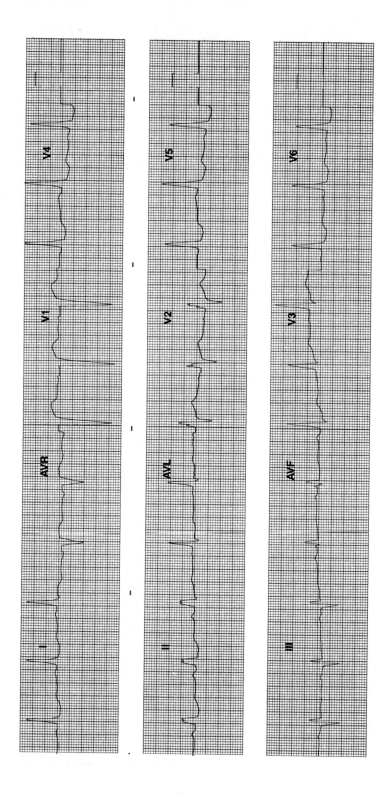

REVIEW ECG 8

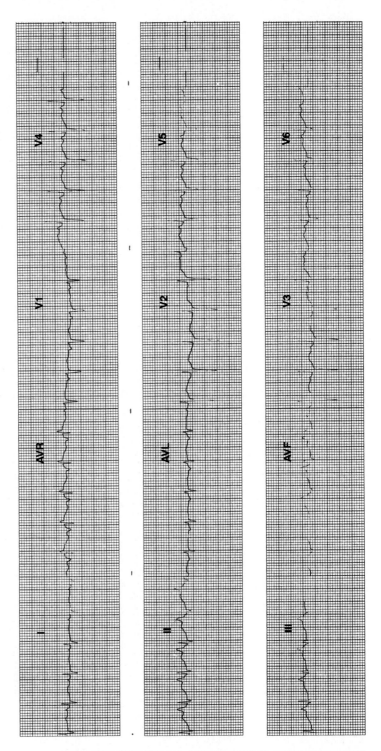

INTRAVENTRICULAR CONDUCTION DISTURBANCES

REVIEW ECG 9

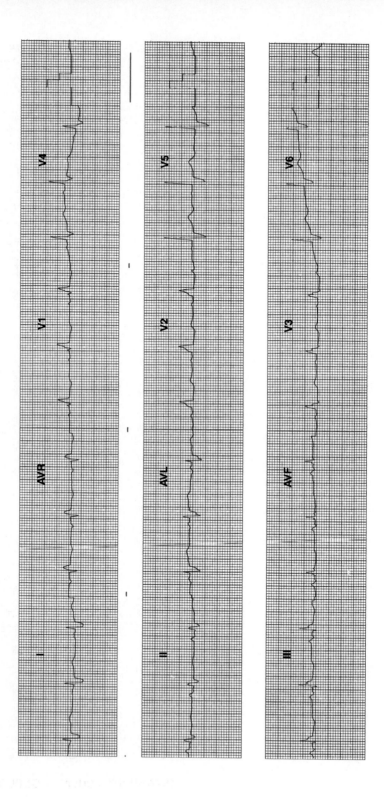

INTRAVENTRICULAR CONDUCTION DISTURBANCES

REVIEW ECG ANSWERS

1. Sinus bradycardia at 43 per minute with left bundle branch block
2. Sinus bradycardia at 57 per minute with left anterior hemiblock
3. Sinus bradycardia at 42 per minute with right bundle branch block and left anterior hemiblock
4. Sinus arrhythmia with nonspecific intraventricular conduction disturbance
5. Sinus rhythm at 69 per minute with left atrial enlargement, right bundle branch block, and left anterior hemiblock
6. Sinus rhythm at 63 per minute with right bundle branch block
7. Sinus rhythm at 65 per minute with first degree AV block and left bundle branch block
8. Sinus tachycardia at 127 per minute with right atrial enlargement and left posterior hemiblock
9. Sinus rhythm at 69 per minute with right bundle branch block and left posterior hemiblock
10. Sinus bradycardia at 53 per minute with right bundle branch block and left posterior hemiblock

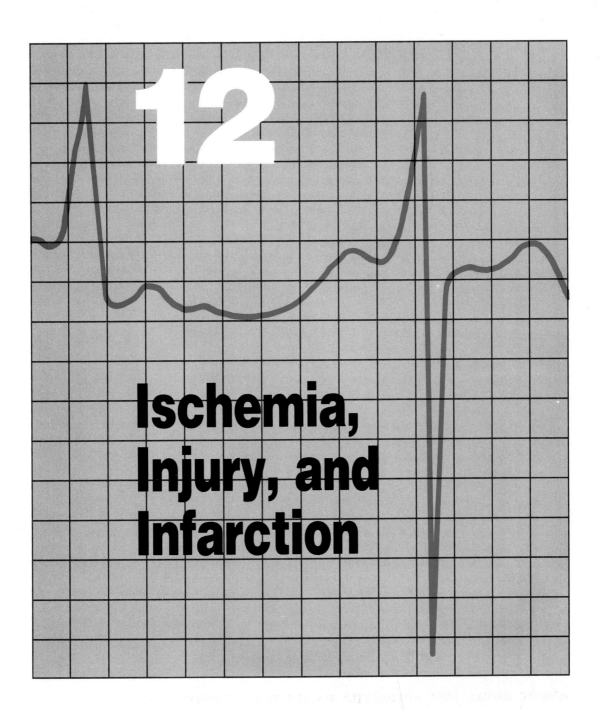

12

Ischemia, Injury, and Infarction

The heart muscle must receive a sufficient blood supply through its own network of arteries, called *coronary arteries*. The two arteries that suply the heart muscle with oxygenated blood are the left and right coronary arteries. The left coronary artery has two major branches—the circumflex branch, which travels to the upper lateral wall of the left ventricle and the left atrium, and the anterior descending branch, which courses down the anterior portion of the heart. The right coronary artery curves around the right ventricle and separates into a variable number of branches.

Variations in the branching pattern of the coronary arteries are common. Left or right coronary artery dominance denotes which artery provides the greatest portion of oxygenated blood to the base of the left ventricle. Sometimes both the left and right coronary arteries have a fairly balanced pattern of distribution of blood, and neither one is considered dominant.

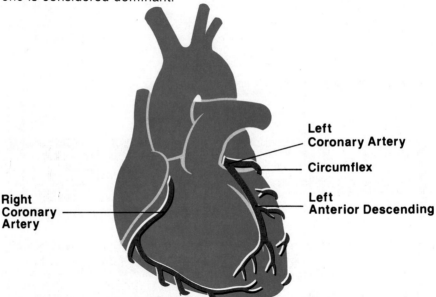

A narrowing of the coronary arteries, often caused by atherosclerosis, results in a diminished blood supply to the heart. During rest, these narrowed coronary arteries may deliver a sufficient blood supply to the heart, but with exertion the rapidly pumping thick left ventricle requires a greater blood supply, and will be the chamber to suffer by reduction in blood flow. Lack of adequate oxygenated blood results in ischemia. If the heart is without a blood supply, injury to the left heart muscle will occur. Finally, if the blood supply is not returned, death of a portion of the left ventricular muscle will occur and is termed *infarction*.

ISCHEMIA

Ischemia is a lack of sufficient oxygenated blood to the left ventricle and is manifested on the ECG by symmetrically inverted T waves or ST depression.

ISCHEMIA

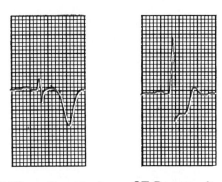

T Wave Inverted   **ST Depression**

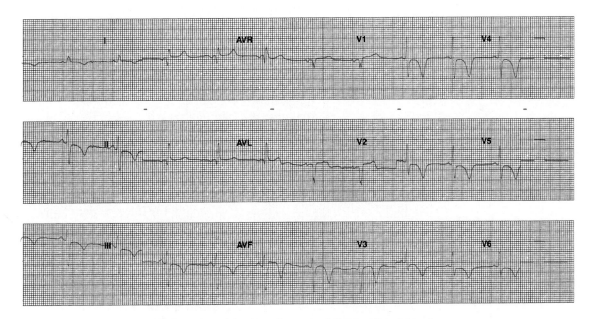

Widespread ischemia noted throughout tracing

ISCHEMIA, INJURY, AND INFARCTION

All the ECG leads should be routinely checked for T wave inversion and ST depression. Remember, T waves are always inverted in aVR and can normally be inverted in lead III and V_1.

NORMAL ECG

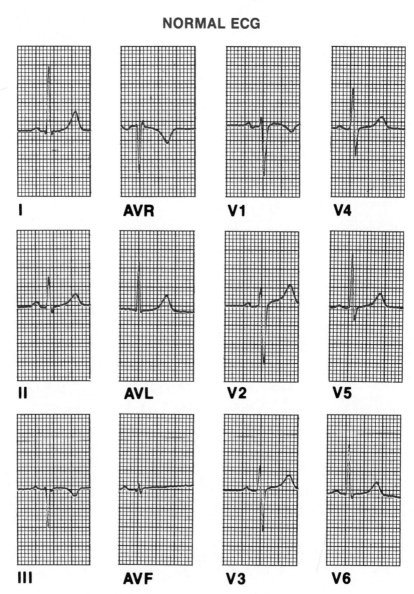

T waves in Lead III and V_1 may be inverted.

INJURY

Injury is a stage beyond ischemia and is manifested on the ECG by ST elevation. Like ischemia, injury is a reversible process, and no permanent damage necessarily occurs. All the leads on an ECG should be routinely checked for ST elevation.

ST SEGMENT ELEVATION

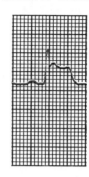

INFARCTION

Infarction is necrosis or death of tissue in a portion of the left ventricular myocardial wall, and follows the stages of ischemia and injury if an adequate blood supply is not returned. Infarction is demonstrated on an ECG by significant Q waves. For Q waves to be considered significant, they must either be .04 second wide or one third the height of the R wave. If neither of these conditions is met, the Q waves are not diagnostic of infarction. Septal Q waves—those normally found in lead I, aVL, V_5, and V_6—represent depolarization of the ventricular septum and are not pathologic.

Q WAVES

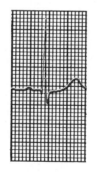

Septal Q Wave

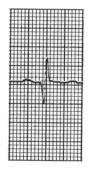

Significant Q Wave

The production of the Q wave of infarction is explained by the use of vectors. The three vectors representing ventricular depolarization in the normal heart are each averages of the electrical forces occurring in the right and left ventricles at a given time. Vector 1 represents septal and early right ventricular activation and is an average of the combined right and left ventricular forces. Vector 2 represents apical activation and is an average of combined electrical forces of the right and left ventricles. Vector 3 denotes left ventricular activation.

VENTRICULAR DEPOLARIZATION

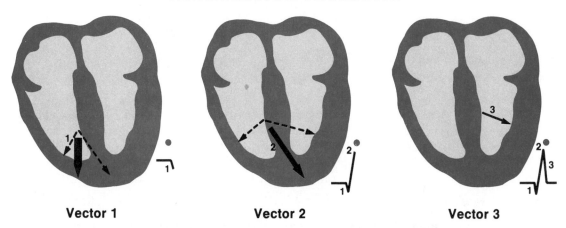

Vector 1   Vector 2   Vector 3

The three vectors representing ventricular depolarization in the normal heart are each averages of the forces occurring in the ventricles at a given time, producing a mean QRS vector moving toward the electrode, and recording a predominantly positive QRS.

With infarction, the electrical forces from the damaged left ventricle are nonexistent, so the electrical forces from the right ventricle are unopposed and a deep and wide Q wave is produced as the electrical forces move away from the electrode during activation of the infarcted area.

ORIGIN OF THE Q WAVE IN INFARCTION

VENTRICULAR DEPOLARIZATION

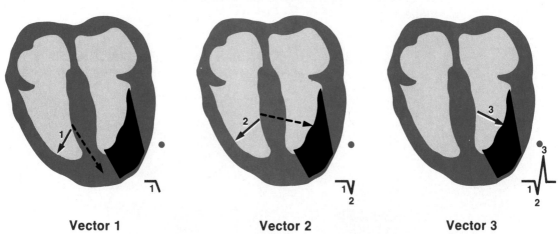

Vector 1   Vector 2   Vector 3

With infarction there are no vectors from the electrically dead area in the left ventricle. The right ventricular vectors are now unopposed and the majority of electrical activity is now traveling away from the electrode, recording a significant Q wave.

When we discuss ischemia, injury, or infarction we are referring to conditions present in the left ventricle. We can be more specific and determine approximately what area of the left ventricle is being affected. The left ventricle is divided into four main locations: anterior, lateral, inferior, and posterior. Leads V_1, V_2, V_3, and V_4 are located over the anterior portion of the left ventricle. Leads I, aVL, V_5, and V_6 are placed over the lateral portion, and leads II, III, and aVF are positioned over the inferior portion of the left ventricle. No leads are placed directly over the posterior aspect of the left ventricle, but by observing the opposite or anterior wall, some determinations can be made.

INFARCT LOCATIONS IN THE LEFT VENTRICLE AND ELECTRODE POSITIONS

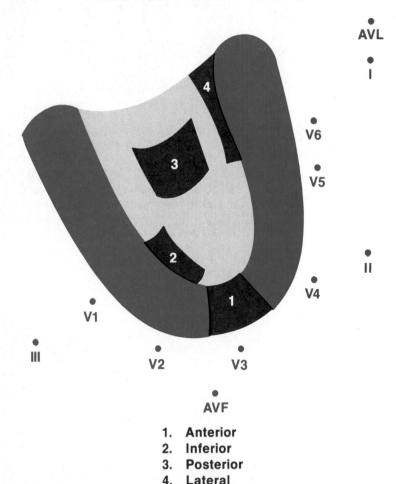

1. **Anterior**
2. **Inferior**
3. **Posterior**
4. **Lateral**

We can classify the infarcted left ventricular muscle electrically into three regions: (1) the region of infarction where the heart muscle is electrically dead and does not conduct any impulses, (2) the region of injury that immediately surrounds the infarcted area and has cell membranes which are never completely polarized, and (3) the region of ischemia in which repolarization is impaired.

INFARCTION, INJURY, AND ISCHEMIA OF THE LEFT VENTRICLE

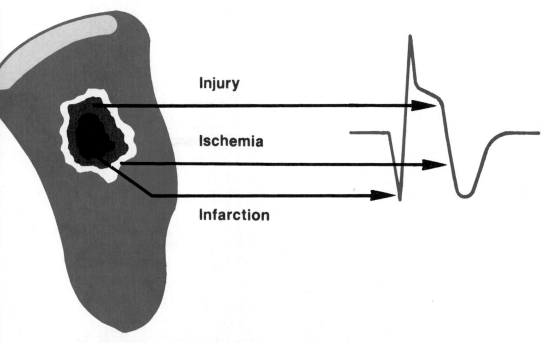

The sequence of stages in the development and evolution of a myocardial infarction usually proceeds as follows:

1. An area of left ventricular muscle is injured and ST elevation occurs in the ECG leads over the injured area.

ST ELEVATION

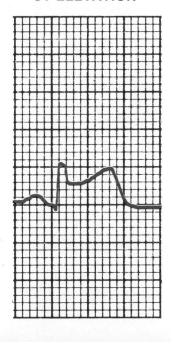

2. Q waves develop in the ECG
   leads over the infarcted area.

Q WAVE

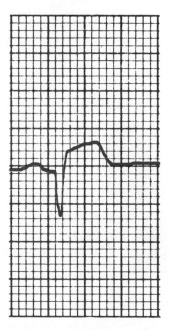

3. T wave inversion occurs in
   the ECG leads over the infarcted area.

**T INVERSION AND
ST ELEVATION REMAINS**

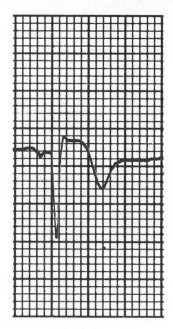

4. ST elevation returns to baseline and T waves remain inverted over the injured myocardium.

ONLY T INVERSION REMAINS

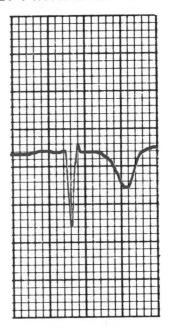

Reciprocal changes in infarction on an ECG are demonstrated by ST depression in the leads opposite the infarcted area.

RECIPROCAL CHANGES OF INFARCTION

INFERIOR INFARCTION

ST DEPRESSION IN LEADS OPPOSITE INFARCTION

| II | III | AVF | I | AVL |

Recuprocal Δ's
ST↓ opposite
injury

We can make a determination about the age of an infarction by examining the ST segment and T waves in the leads over the infarcted area. If the ST segments are elevated, the infarction is probably acute. If the ST segments are at baseline and the T waves are inverted, we might conclude that an infarction is present with an age indeterminate. On the other hand, if the ST segments are at baseline and the T waves are upright, we might conclude that the infarction is old. It is often difficult to make exact determinations of infarction age from isolated ECGs.

ACUTE INFARCTION   **INFARCTION, AGE INDETERMINATE**   **OLD INFARCTION**

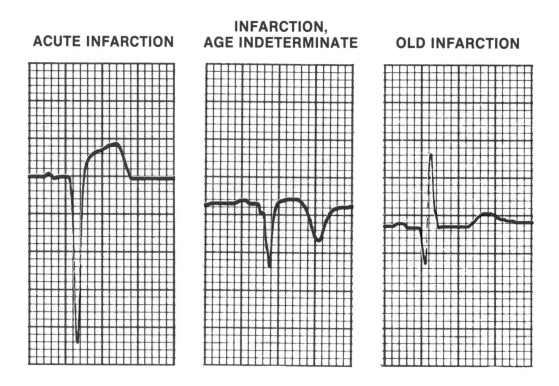

Infarction can be determined by identifying significant Q waves in at least two ECG leads for each infarct location or by noting loss of R wave potential.

Anterior Infarction. Q waves in V_1, V_2, V_3, or V_4

ANTERIOR INFARCTION

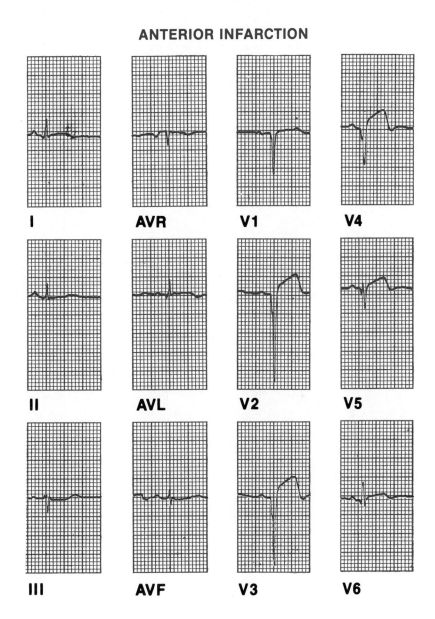

I	AVR	V1	V4
II	AVL	V2	V5
III	AVF	V3	V6

Anterior Septal Infarction. Q waves in V_1 and V_2 only or poor R wave progression in V_1 and V_2

ANTERIOR SEPTAL INFARCTION

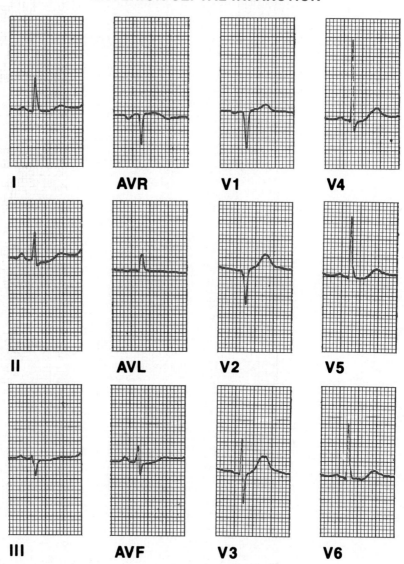

ANTERIOR SEPTAL INFARCTION

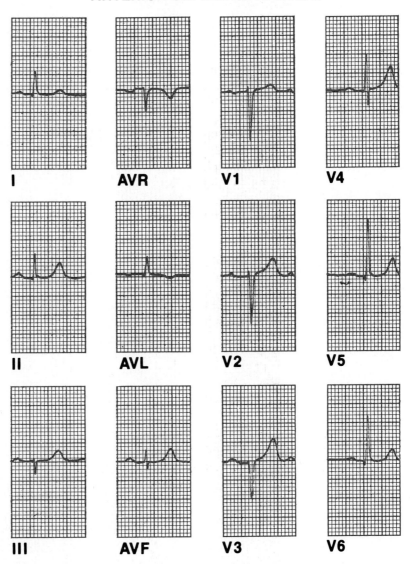

Q waves in V_1 and V_2 or poor R wave progression may also be caused by left ventricular hypertrophy. Always consider left ventricular hypertrophy to be the source of these abnormalities, but do not rule out the possibility of an anterior septal myocardial infarction.

ISCHEMIA, INJURY, AND INFARCTION

Lateral Infarction. Q waves in I, aVL, V_5, or V_6

LATERAL INFARCTION

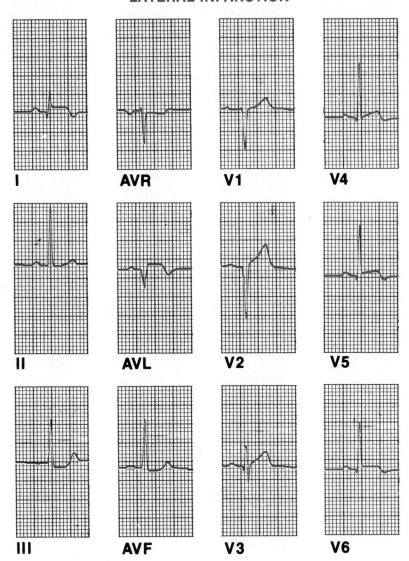

I	AVR	V1	V4
II	AVL	V2	V5
III	AVF	V3	V6

Inferior Infarction. Q waves in II, III, or aVF

INFERIOR INFARCTION

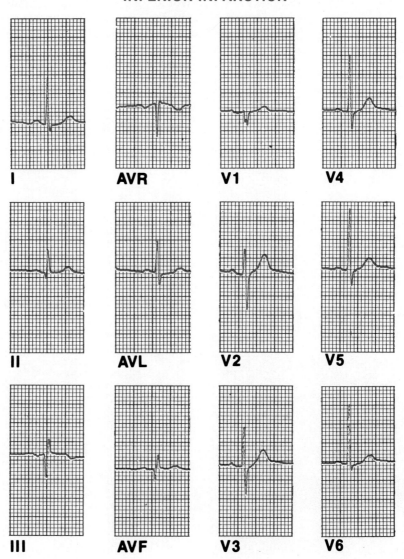

I   AVR   V1   V4

II   AVL   V2   V5

III   AVF   V3   V6

Posterior Infarction. Tall R waves in V_1 and V_2, often accompanied by tall T waves. A posterior infarction is recognized by using the ECG leads on the opposite or anterior wall. Instead of inspecting for significant Q waves, you would inspect for the opposite effect or tall R waves. An acute posterior infarction would have depressed rather than elevated ST segments. It is difficult to determine with accuracy whether a posterior infarction is present or whether the tall R waves are a normal variant. Always suspect a posterior infarction when tall R waves are present in V_1 and V_2, accompanied by an inferior infarction.

POSTERIOR INFARCTION

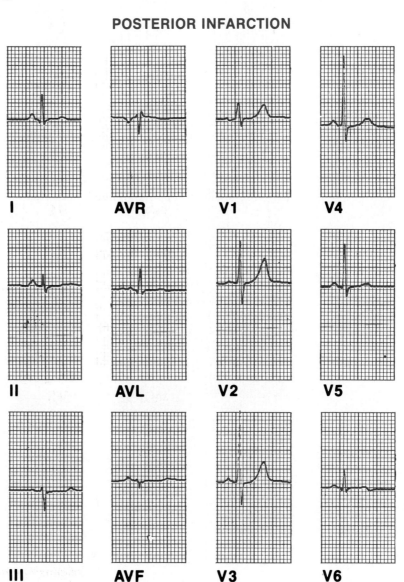

I	AVR	V1	V4
II	AVL	V2	V5
III	AVF	V3	V6

208

INFERIOR POSTERIOR INFARCTION

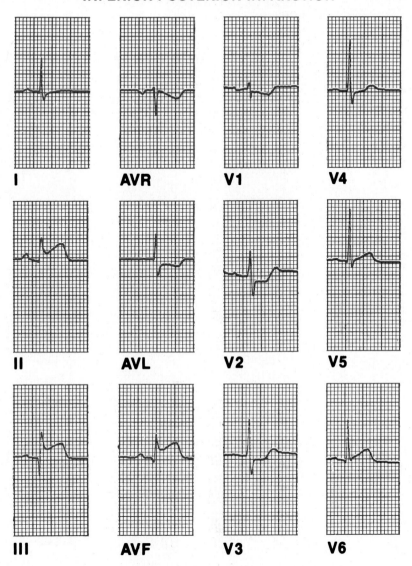

Infarctions can occur either as isolated events or in various combinations.

ANTERIOR LATERAL INFARCTION

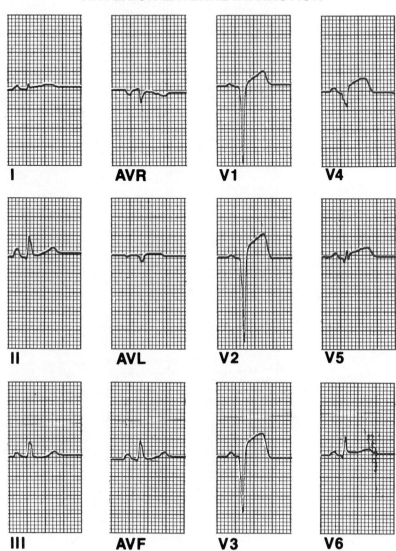

ANTERIOR, LATERAL, AND INFERIOR INFARCTION

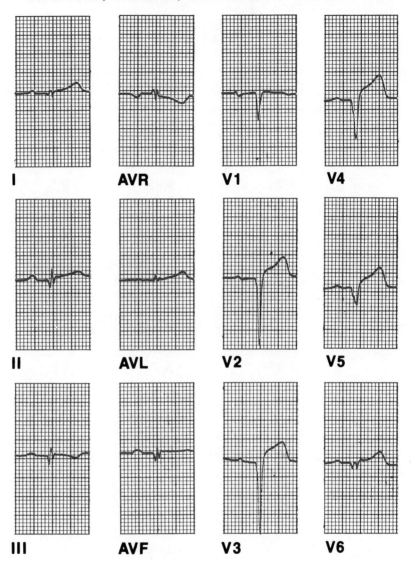

I	AVR	V1	V4
II	AVL	V2	V5
III	AVF	V3	V6

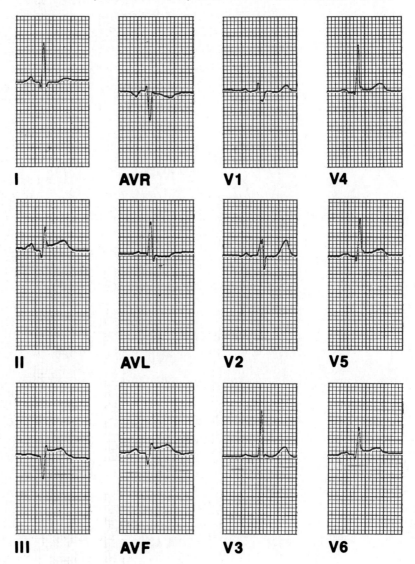

I	AVR	V1	V4
II	AVL	V2	V5
III	AVF	V3	V6

Myocardial infarction should not be diagnosed in the presence of left bundle branch block. The right ventricle depolarizes before the left ventricle in left bundle branch block, so any Q wave signifying infarction would be buried in the QRS rather than appearing at the beginning of the complex.

DO NOT DIAGNOSE INFARCTION IN THE PRESENCE OF LEFT BUNDLE BRANCH BLOCK

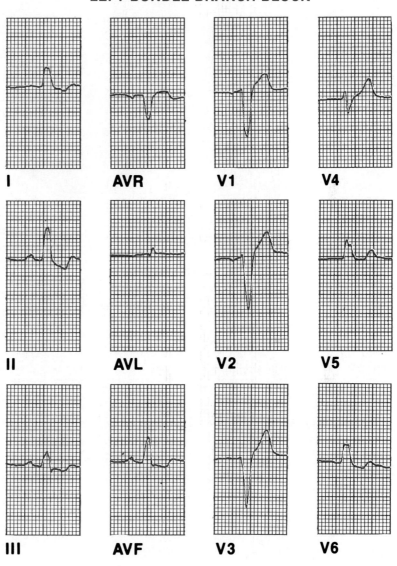

ISCHEMIA, INJURY, AND INFARCTION

ANTERIOR INFARCTION

ECG Leads to Check for Anterior Infarction

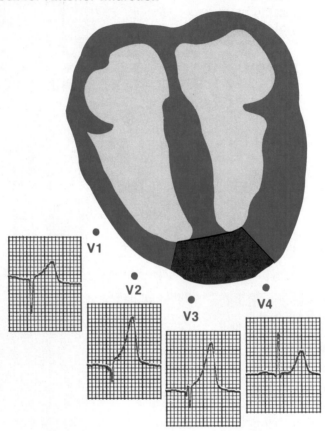

Criterion

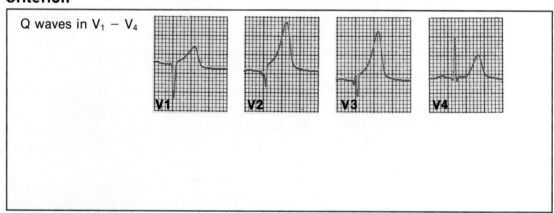

Q waves in $V_1 - V_4$

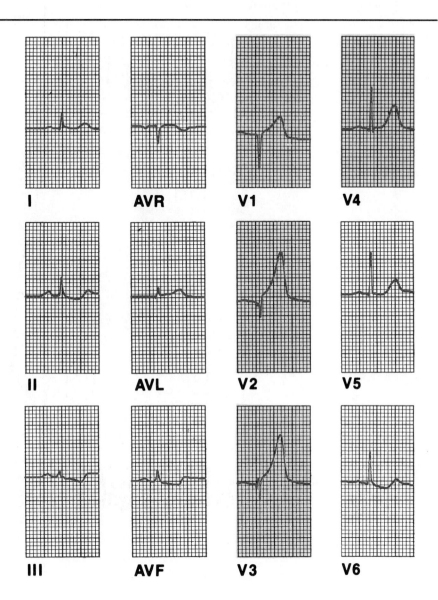

I AVR V1 V4

II AVL V2 V5

III AVF V3 V6

ISCHEMIA, INJURY, AND INFARCTION

ANTERIOR SEPTAL INFARCTION

ECG Leads to Check for Anterior Septal Infarction

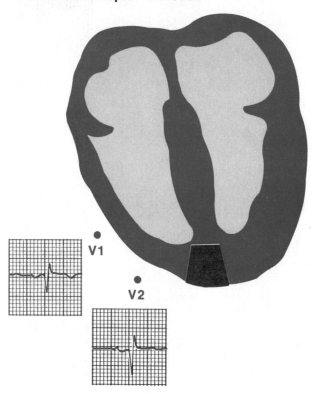

Criterion

Q waves in V_1 and V_2
   or
Poor R wave progression in V_1 and V_2

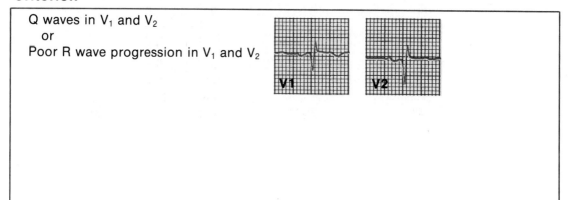

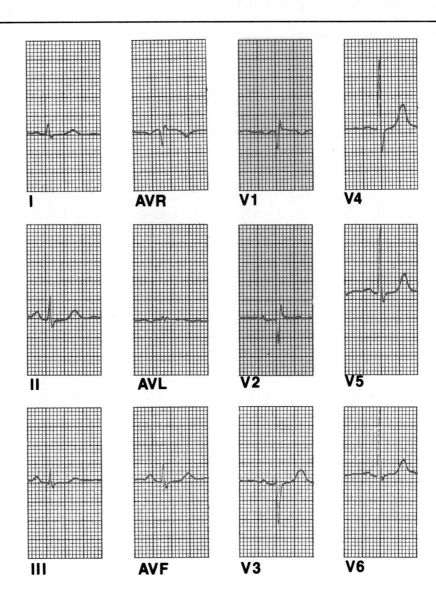

I AVR V1 V4

II AVL V2 V5

III AVF V3 V6

ISCHEMIA, INJURY, AND INFARCTION

ECG Leads to Check for Lateral Infarction

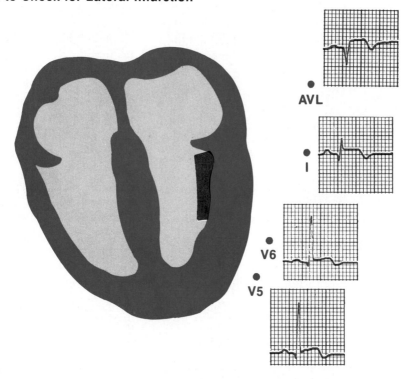

Criterion

Q waves in I, aVL, V_5, and V_6

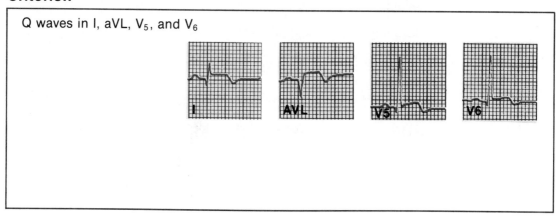

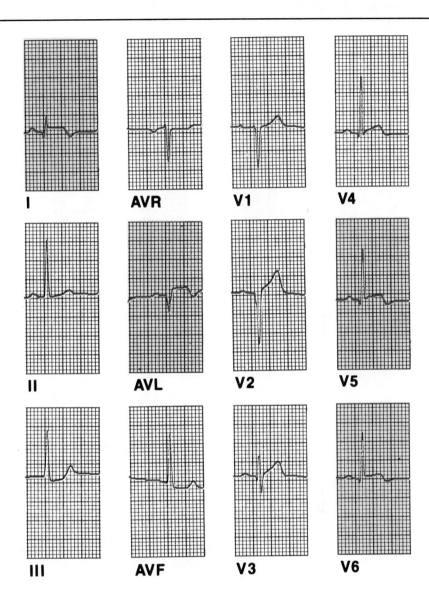

I AVR V1 V4

II AVL V2 V5

III AVF V3 V6

INFERIOR INFARCTION

ECG Leads to Check for Inferior Infarction

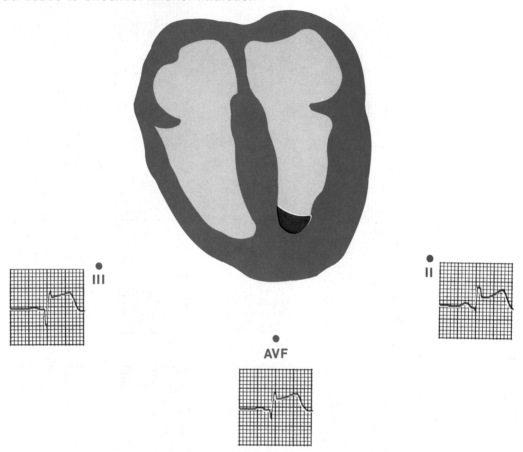

Criterion

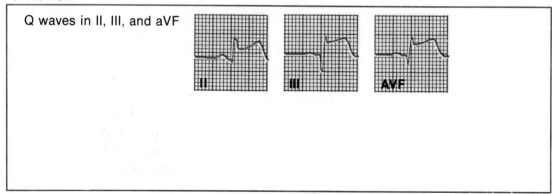

Q waves in II, III, and aVF

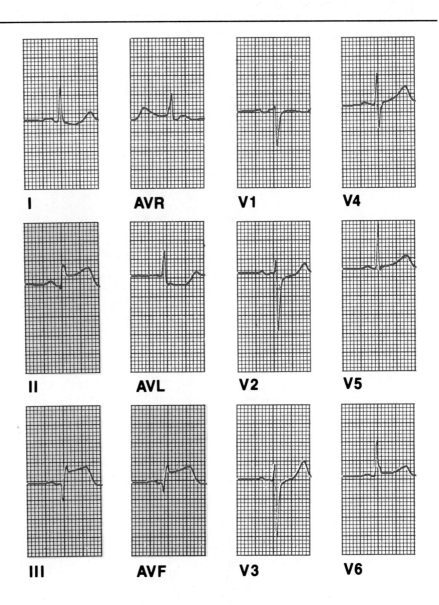

I AVR V1 V4

II AVL V2 V5

III AVF V3 V6

ISCHEMIA, INJURY, AND INFARCTION

POSTERIOR INFARCTION

ECG Leads to Check for Posterior Infarction

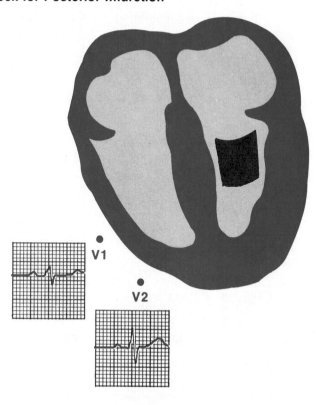

Criterion

Tall R waves in V_1 and V_2 often accompanied by tall T waves

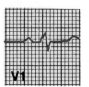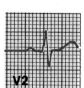

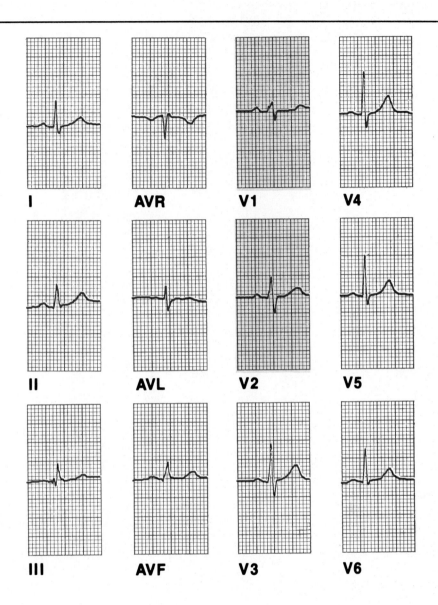

I   AVR   V1   V4

II   AVL   V2   V5

III   AVF   V3   V6

ISCHEMIA, INJURY, AND INFARCTION

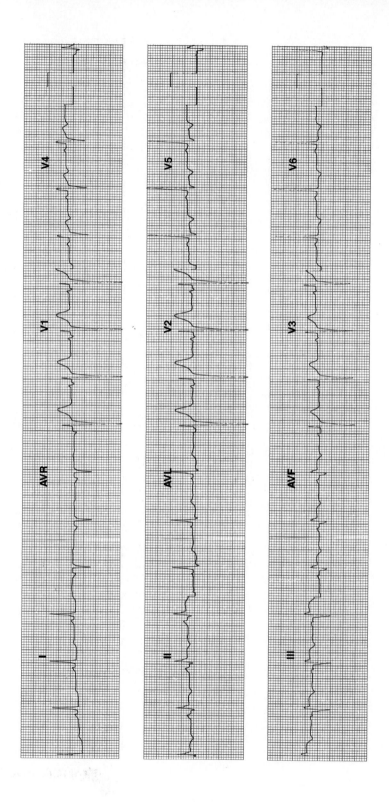

REVIEW ECG 2

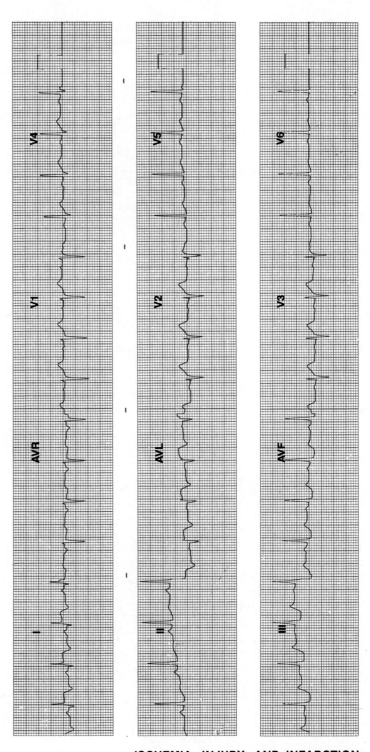

ISCHEMIA, INJURY, AND INFARCTION

225

REVIEW ECG 3

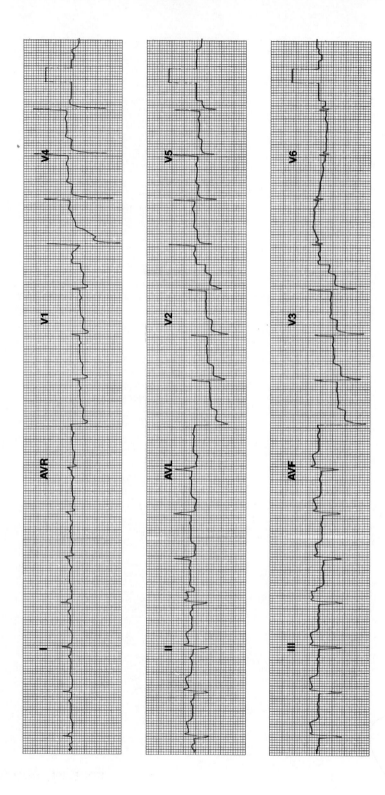

REVIEW ECG 4

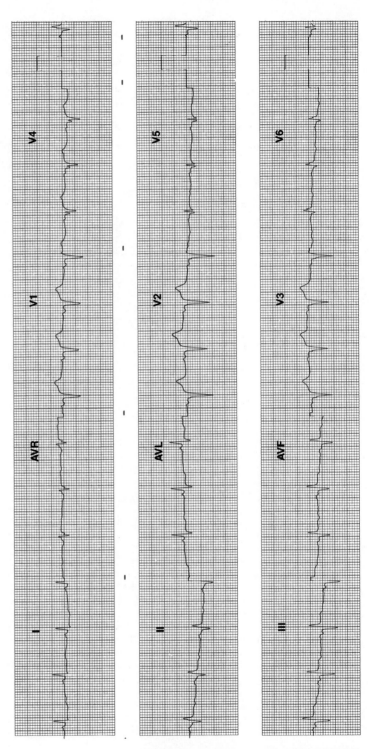

ISCHEMIA, INJURY, AND INFARCTION

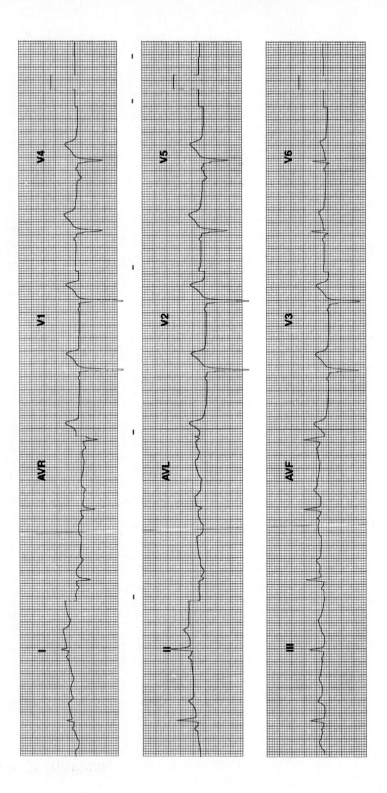

REVIEW ECG 6

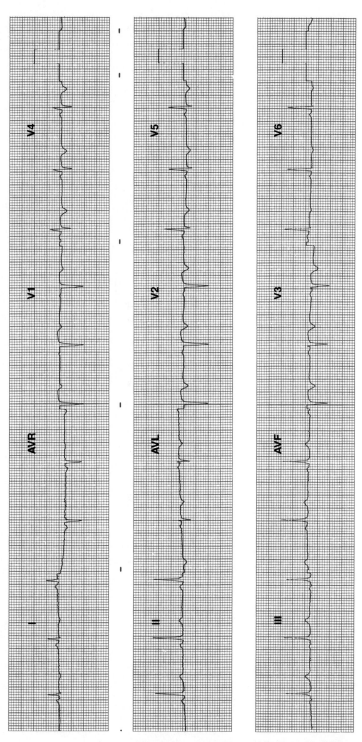

ISCHEMIA, INJURY, AND INFARCTION

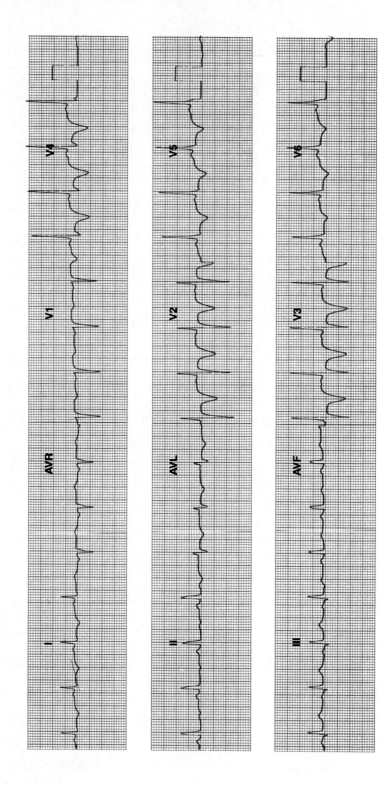

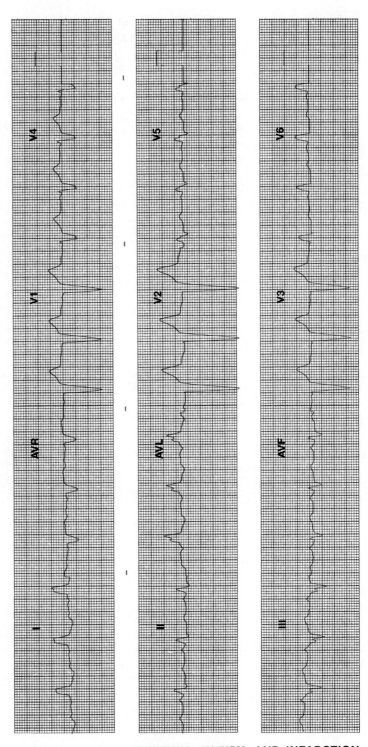

ISCHEMIA, INJURY, AND INFARCTION

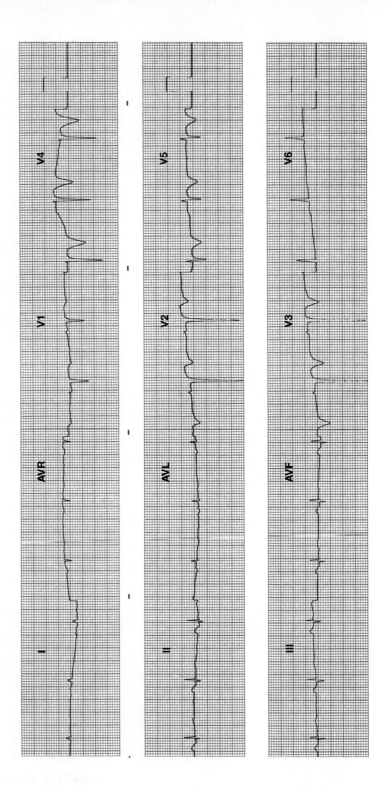

REVIEW ECG 10

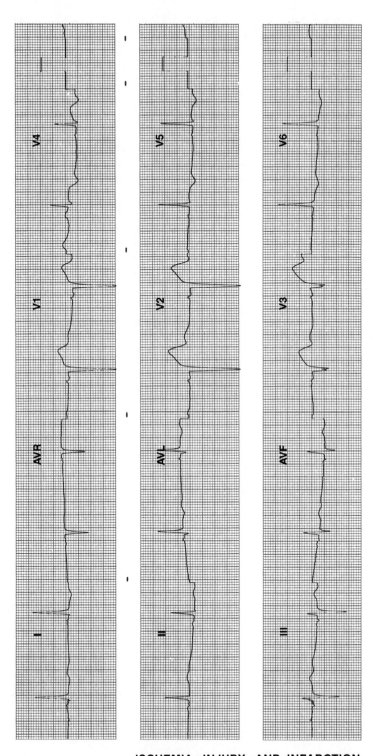

ISCHEMIA, INJURY, AND INFARCTION

REVIEW ECG ANSWERS

1. Sinus rhythm at 82 per minute with left atrial enlargement, left ventricular hypertrophy, and an acute inferior infarction
2. Sinus rhythm at 95 per minute with an acute lateral infarction
3. Sinus rhythm at 86 per minute with acute inferior and posterior infarctions
4. Sinus rhythm at 84 per minute with acute anterior, lateral, and inferior infarctions
5. Sinus bradycardia at 55 per minute with acute anterior and lateral infarctions
6. Sinus rhythm at 66 per minute with an anteroseptal infarction and lateral T wave abnormalities, age indeterminate
7. Sinus rhythm at 85 per minute with anterolateral ischemia
8. Sinus rhythm at 77 per minute with left bundle branch block
9. Sinus rhythm at 64 per minute with an old inferior infarction and an anterior infarction, age indeterminate
10. Sinus bradycardia at 47 per minute with left ventricular hypertrophy and an acute anterior infarction

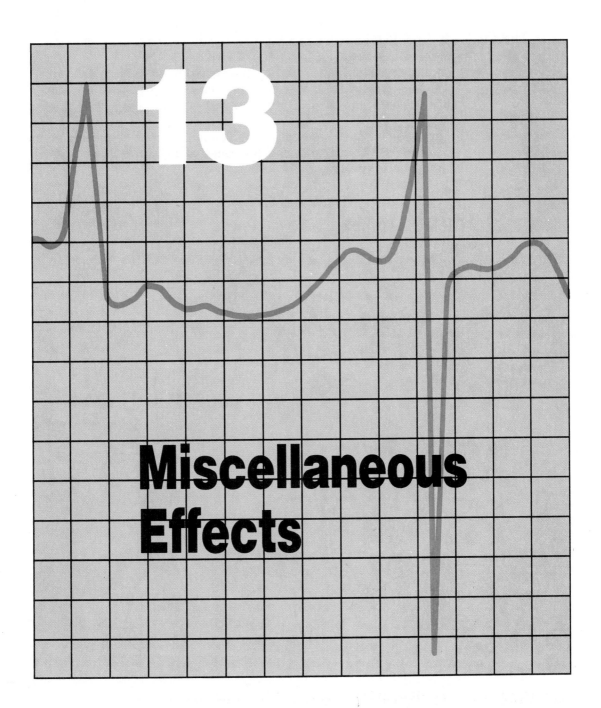

13

Miscellaneous Effects

This chapter discusses how ECGs may suggest electrolyte disturbances, demonstrate drug effects, pericarditis, dextrocardia, and early repolarization. An overview of pediatric ECGs is also included.

ELECTROLYTE DISTURBANCES

Electrolyte disturbances are only suggested on an ECG by ST-T abnormalities. To make a correct diagnosis, a clinical evaluation must be correlated with the ECG results.

Hypokalemia. A lowered potassium concentration is suggested on an ECG by a flat T wave and the occurrence of a U wave. ST depression is sometimes present.

U WAVE

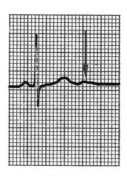

HYPOKALEMIA

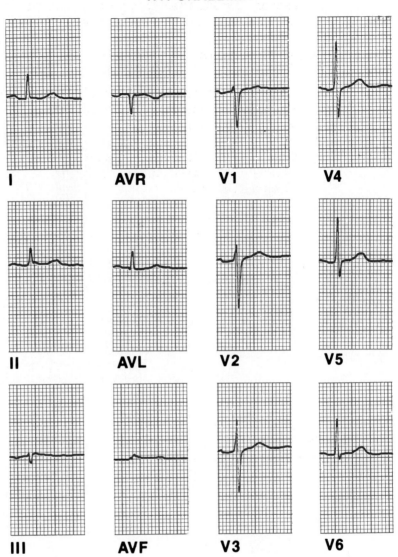

I   AVR   V1   V4

II   AVL   V2   V5

III   AVF   V3   V6

Hyperkalemia. An elevated serum potassium level is indicated on the ECG by peaked or tent-shaped T waves.

TENT-SHAPED T WAVE

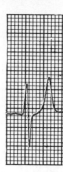

HYPERKALEMIA

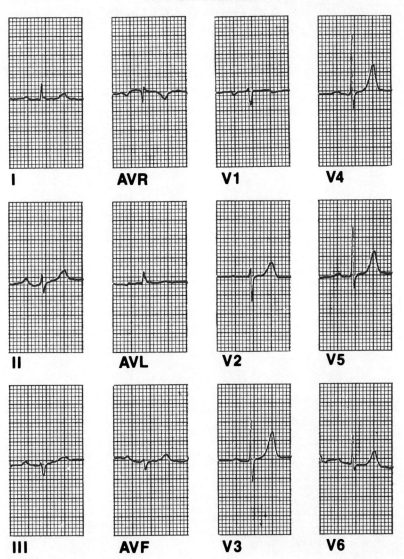

I   AVR   V1   V4

II   AVL   V2   V5

III   AVF   V3   V6

MISCELLANEOUS EFFECTS

Hypocalcemia. A reduced calcium concentration is reflected on the ECG by a prolonged QT interval, which is a result of prolongation of the ST segment.

PROLONGED ST SEGMENT

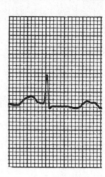

HYPOCALCEMIA

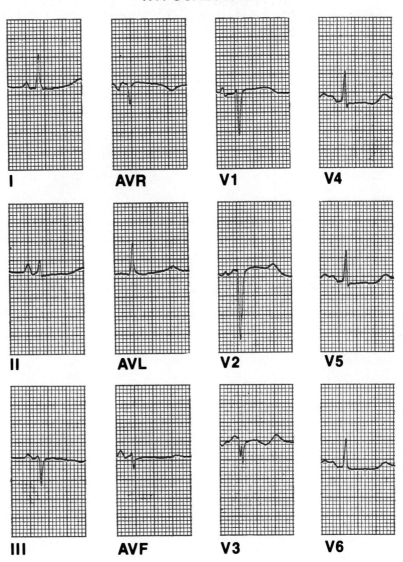

I AVR V1 V4

II AVL V2 V5

III AVF V3 V6

Hypercalcemia. An elevation of the serum calcium level is displayed on the ECG by a shortened QT interval, which is due to a short or absent ST segment.

SHORT ST SEGMENT

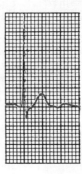

HYPERCALCEMIA

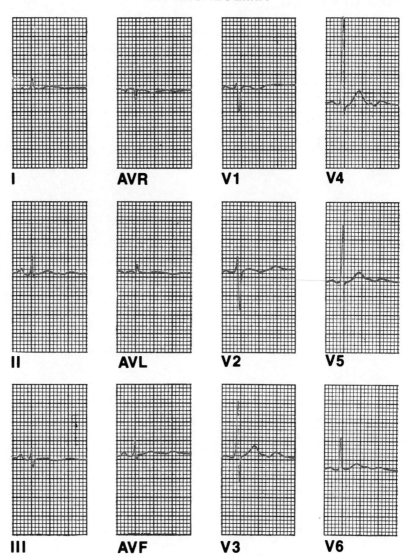

I   AVR   V1   V4

II   AVL   V2   V5

III   AVF   V3   V6

MISCELLANEOUS EFFECTS

DRUG EFFECTS

Digitalis. Digitalis causes a characteristic downward sloping or scooping of the ST segment and a flattened or inverted T wave. The ST-T changes are usually seen in the leads with tall R waves, and these changes often mask ischemic changes.

ST SCOOPING

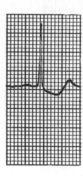

DIGITALIS EFFECT

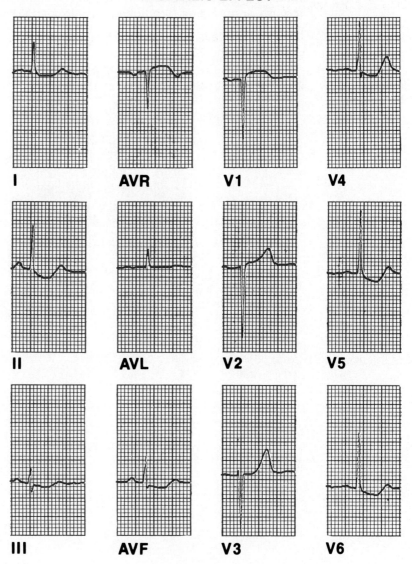

I AVR V1 V4

II AVL V2 V5

III AVF V3 V6

Quinidine. The repolarization time of the ventricles is increased with the use of quinidine, producing a prolonged QT interval and ST-T abnormalities.

MARKED QT PROLONGATION

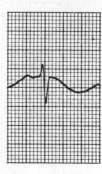

QUINIDINE EFFECT

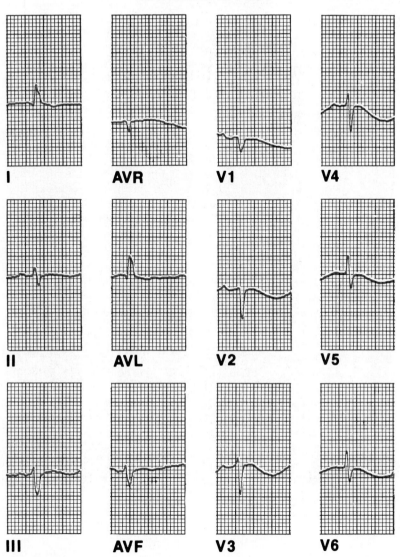

I AVR V1 V4

II AVL V2 V5

III AVF V3 V6

PERICARDITIS

Pericarditis is an inflammation of the pericardial sac surrounding the heart. The ECG demonstrates ST segment elevation, which assumes a concave curvature and subsequent T wave inversion.

PERICARDITIS

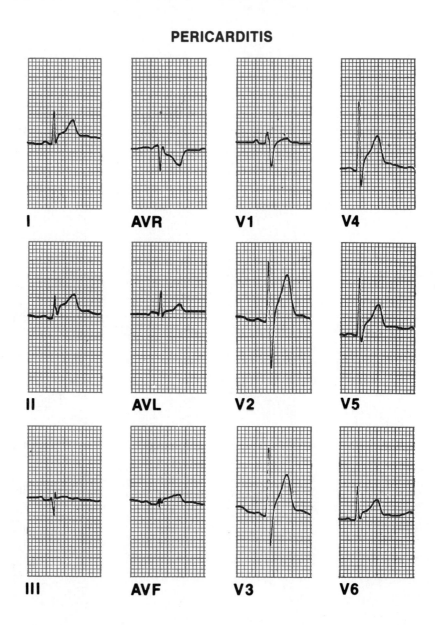

EARLY REPOLARIZATION

Early repolarization is characterized by ST segment elevation, especially in the left precordial leads—V_4, V_5, and V_6. The etiology for early repolarization is not entirely understood, but it is considered to be a normal variant.

EARLY REPOLARIZATION

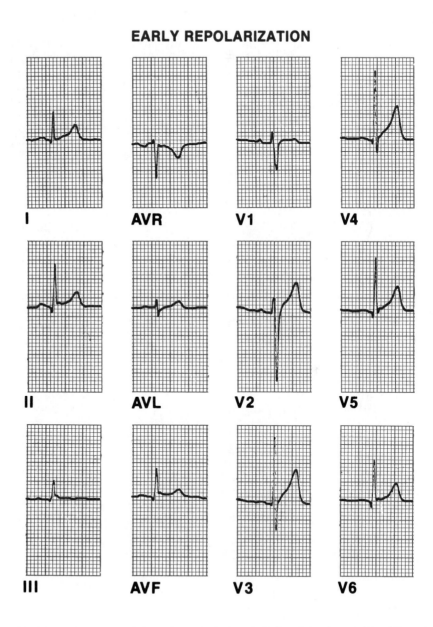

I   AVR   V1   V4

II   AVL   V2   V5

III   AVF   V3   V6

Making a distinction between pericarditis and early repolarization is best accomplished with the use of serial ECGs. The ST elevation of early repolarization remains unaffected by time, but the ST elevation of pericarditis eventually normalizes, and subsequent T wave inversion will often occur.

DEXTROCARDIA

Dextrocardia is demonstrated by complete transposition of the heart to the right side of the chest cavity. The ECG illustrates a mirror image of a normal ECG, resembling a tracing recorded with reversed arm leads and chest leads positioned on the wrong side of the chest cavity. The P, QRS, and T waves will be inverted in lead I and upright in aVR. R wave progression will be reversed, and the tallest R wave will occur in V_1, which will be the lead nearest the heart, and as the chest leads move away from the heart a total loss of R waves will occur.

DEXTROCARDIA

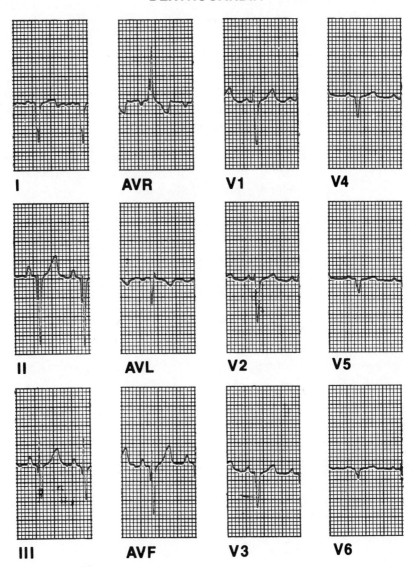

I   AVR   V1   V4

II   AVL   V2   V5

III   AVF   V3   V6

PEDIATRIC ECGS

At birth, the right ventricle is as thick or thicker than the left, and the ECG demonstrates right ventricular hypertrophy. In utero, the resistance to flow in the systemic circulation is lower than in the pulmonary vascular bed, so the work of the right ventricle is much greater than that of the left. After birth, right ventricular pressure decreases and systemic resistance increases, and the left ventricle becomes thicker than the right.

Right axis deviation is also observed and may remain up to one year or more. T waves are normally inverted in V_1 through V_3 and are occasionally further leftward.

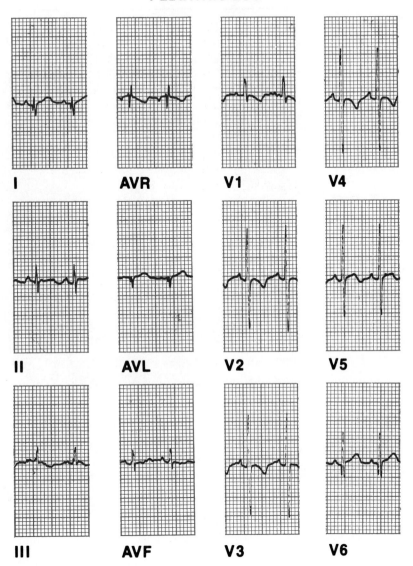

I AVR V1 V4

II AVL V2 V5

III AVF V3 V6

MISCELLANEOUS EFFECTS

HYPOKALEMIA

Check All ECG Leads for Hypokalemia

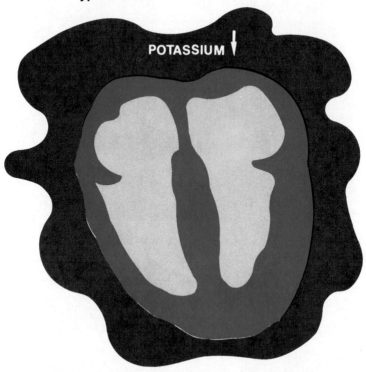

Criterion

Presence of a U wave and a flattened T wave

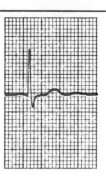

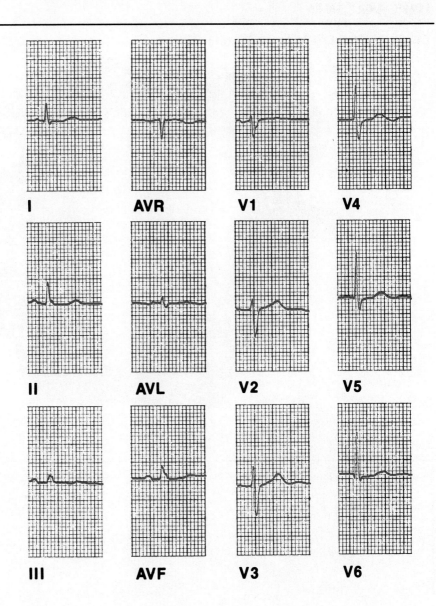

I   AVR   V1   V4

II   AVL   V2   V5

III   AVF   V3   V6

HYPERKALEMIA

Check All ECG Leads for Hyperkalemia

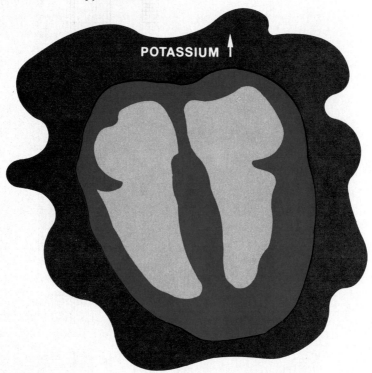

Criterion

Peaked and tent-shaped T waves

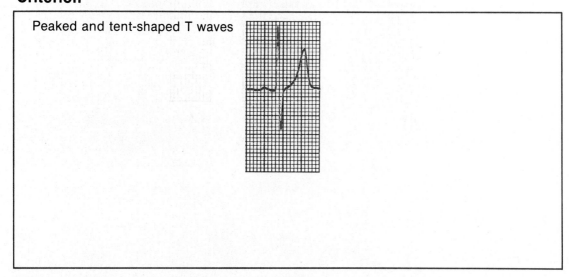

HOW TO QUICKLY AND ACCURATELY MASTER ECG INTERPRETATION

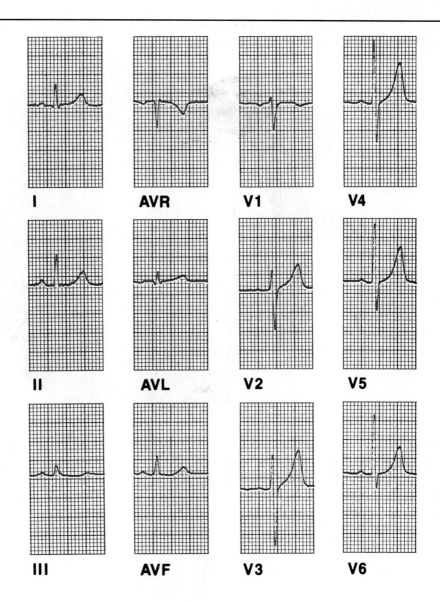

I AVR V1 V4

II AVL V2 V5

III AVF V3 V6

HYPOCALCEMIA

Check All ECG Leads for Hypocalcemia

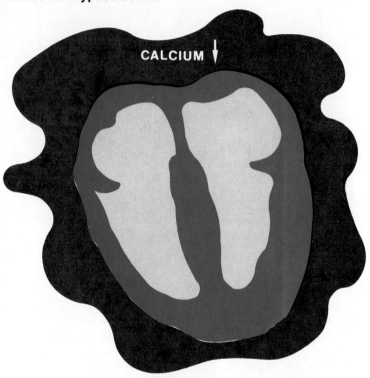

Criterion

Prolongation of the ST segment

HOW TO QUICKLY AND ACCURATELY MASTER ECG INTERPRETATION

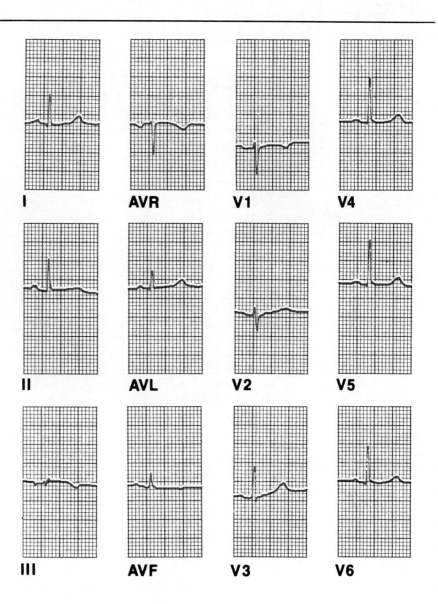

I AVR V1 V4

II AVL V2 V5

III AVF V3 V6

HYPERCALCEMIA

Check All ECG Leads for Hypercalcemia

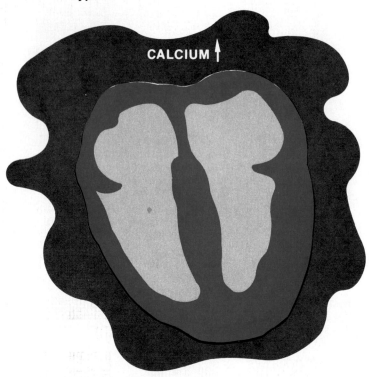

CALCIUM ↑

Criterion

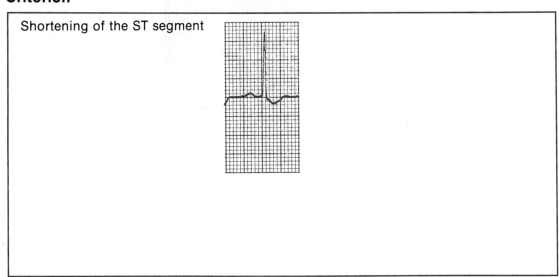

Shortening of the ST segment

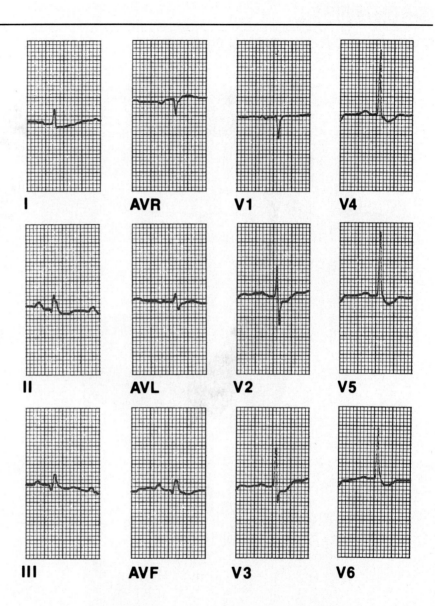

I AVR V1 V4

II AVL V2 V5

III AVF V3 V6

DIGITALIS EFFECT

ECG Leads to Check for Digitalis Effect

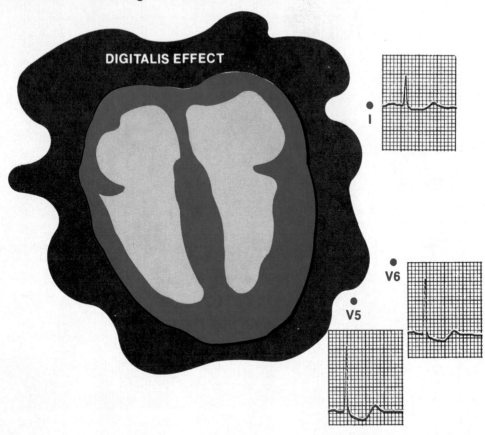

Criterion

Downward sloping or scooping of the ST segment and a flattened or inverted T wave, best seen in leads with tall R waves

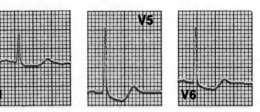

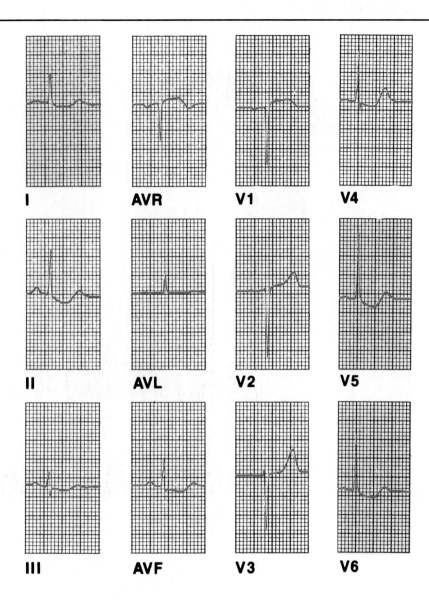

I	AVR	V1	V4
II	AVL	V2	V5
III	AVF	V3	V6

QUINIDINE EFFECT

Check All ECG Leads for Quinidine Effect

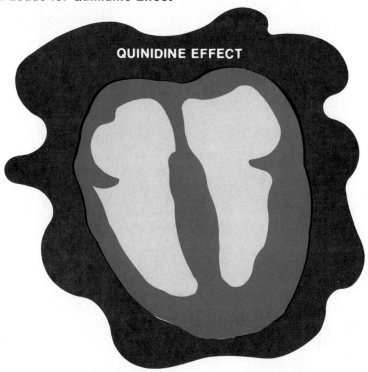

QUINIDINE EFFECT

Criterion

Prolonged QT interval and ST-T abnormalities

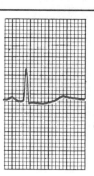

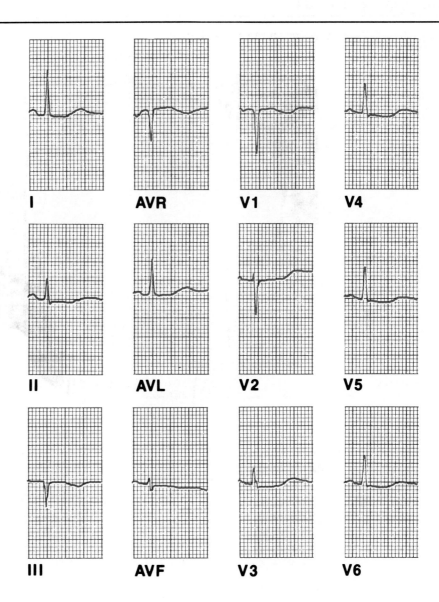

I AVR V1 V4

II AVL V2 V5

III AVF V3 V6

Check All ECG Leads for Pericarditis

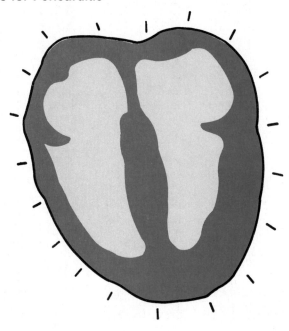

Criterion

ST segment elevation that assumes a concave curvature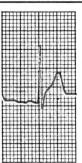

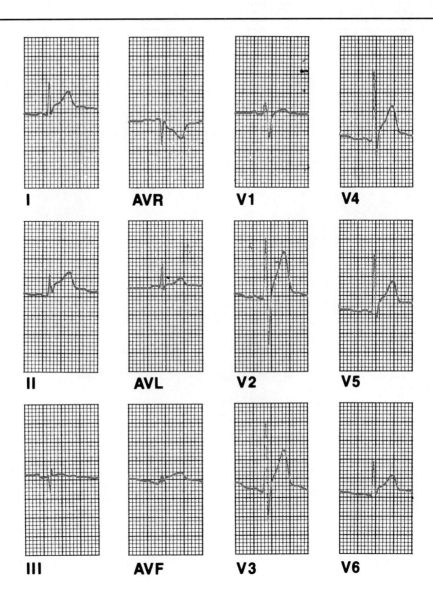

I   AVR   V1   V4

II   AVL   V2   V5

III   AVF   V3   V6

EARLY REPOLARIZATION

ECG Leads to Check for Early Repolarization

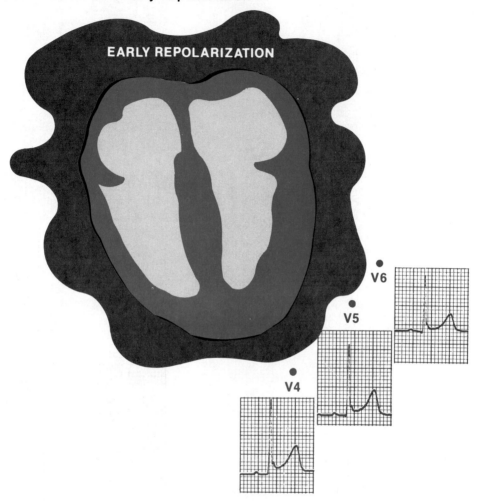

Criterion

ST segment elevation, especially in V_4, V_5, and V_6

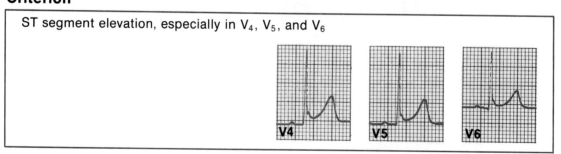

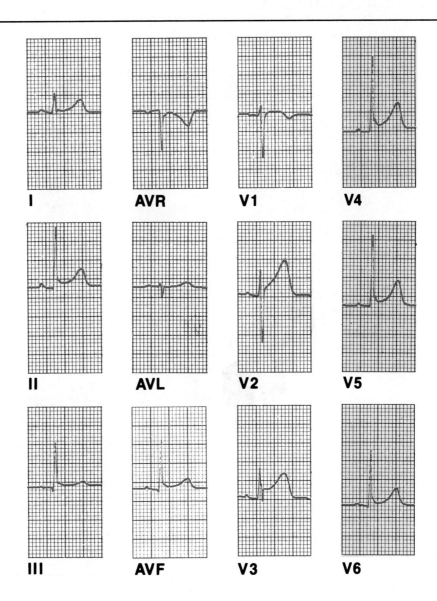

I   AVR   V1   V4

II   AVL   V2   V5

III   AVF   V3   V6

DEXTROCARDIA

ECG Leads to Check for Dextrocardia

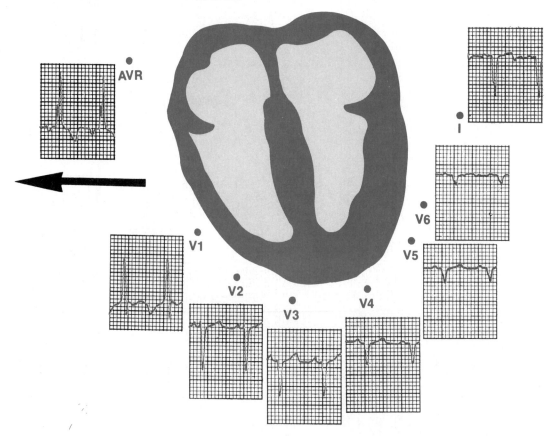

Criteria

1. P, QRS, and T waves often inverted in lead I
2. P, QRS, and T waves upright in aVR

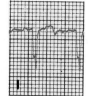 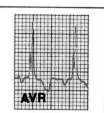

3. R wave progression will be reversed—the tallest R wave occurs in V_1 and will become progressively smaller as the chest leads move away from the heart.

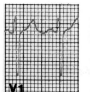 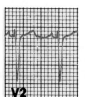 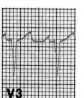 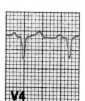 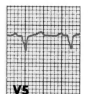 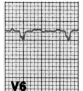

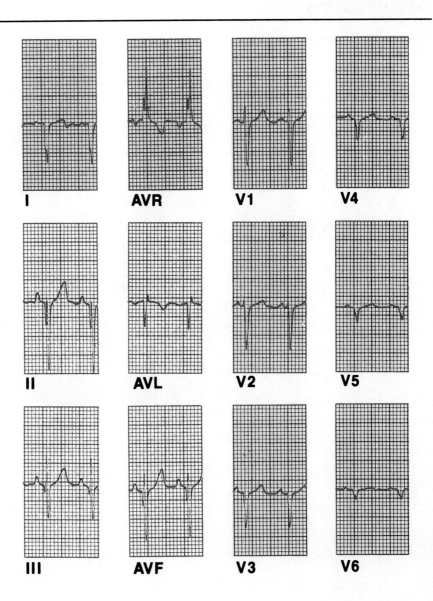

I AVR V1 V4

II AVL V2 V5

III AVF V3 V6

PEDIATRIC ECGS

ECG Leads to Check for Pediatric ECG

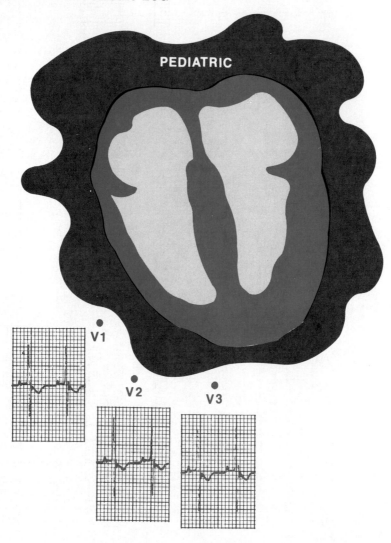

Criteria

1. Right axis deviation is present.

2. T waves may be inverted in V_1, V_2, and V_3.

3. Sinus tachycardia is a normal manifestation in infancy.

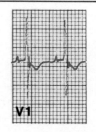
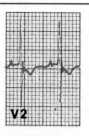
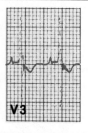

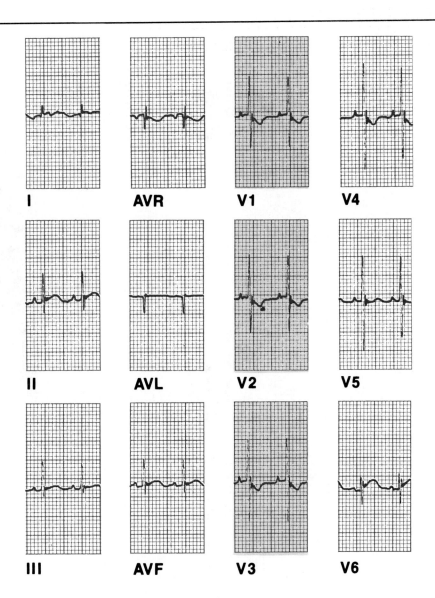

I   AVR   V1   V4

II   AVL   V2   V5

III   AVF   V3   V6

MISCELLANEOUS EFFECTS

273

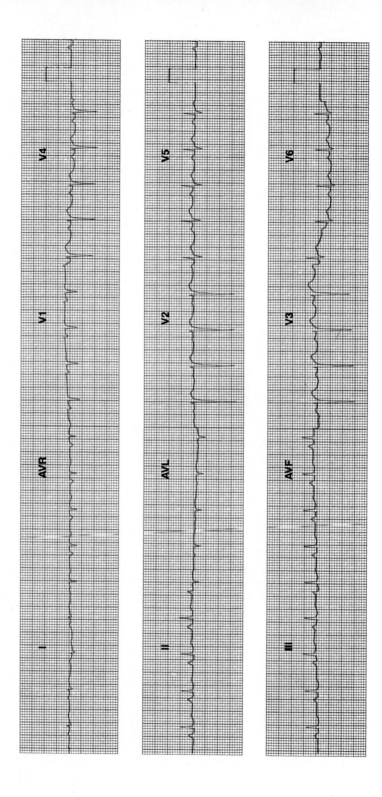

REVIEW ECG 2

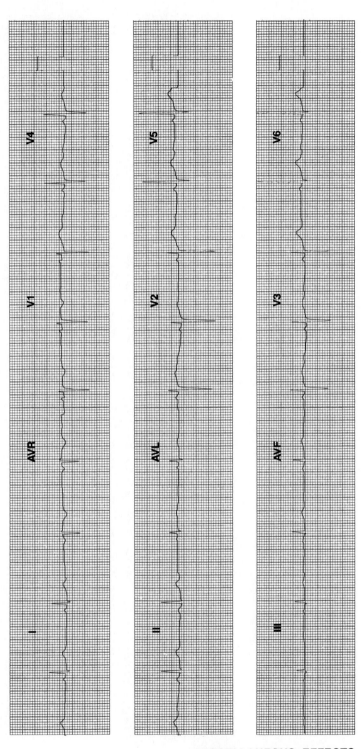

MISCELLANEOUS EFFECTS

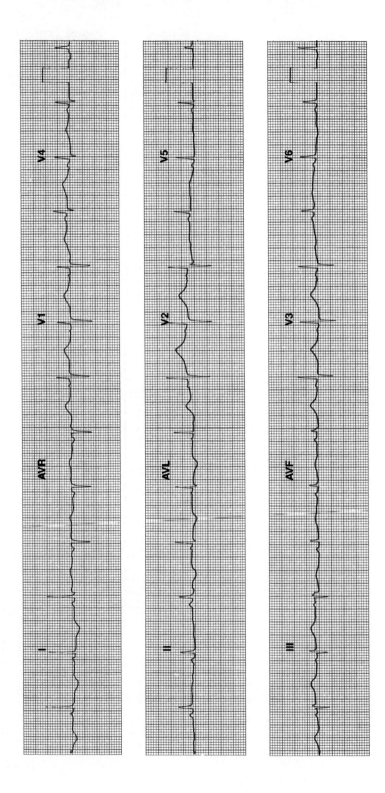

REVIEW ECG 4

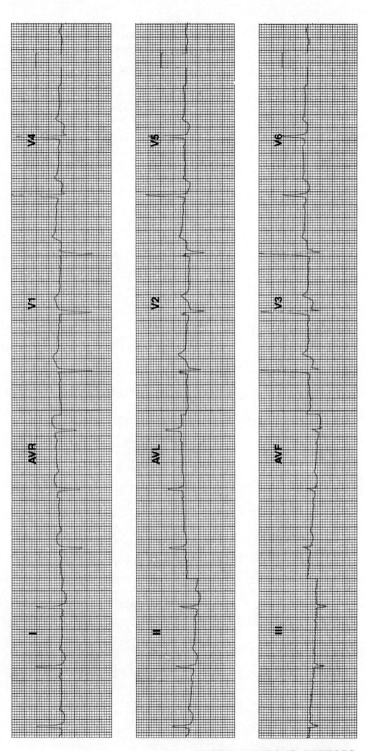

MISCELLANEOUS EFFECTS

277

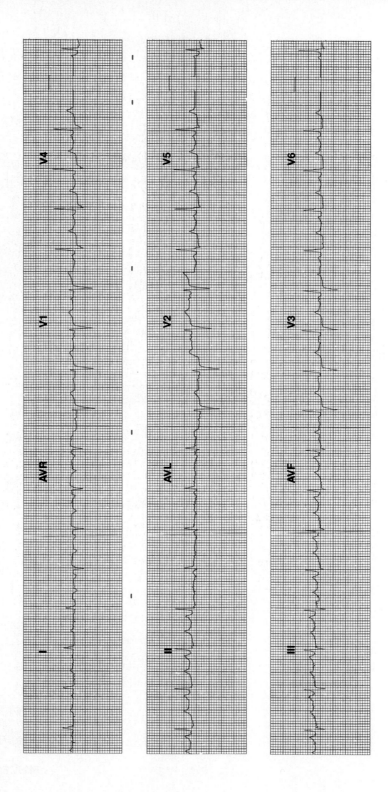

REVIEW ECG 6

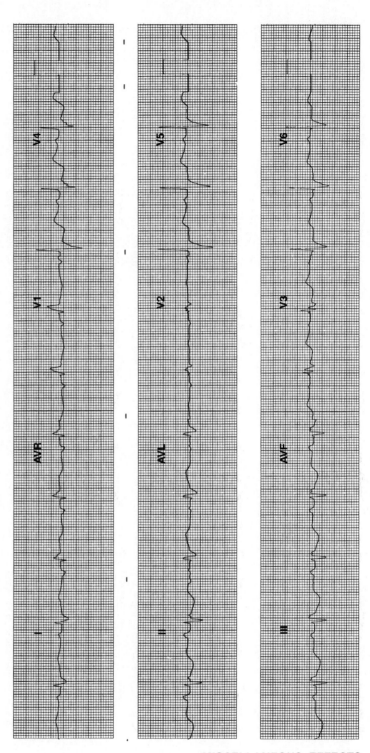

MISCELLANEOUS EFFECTS

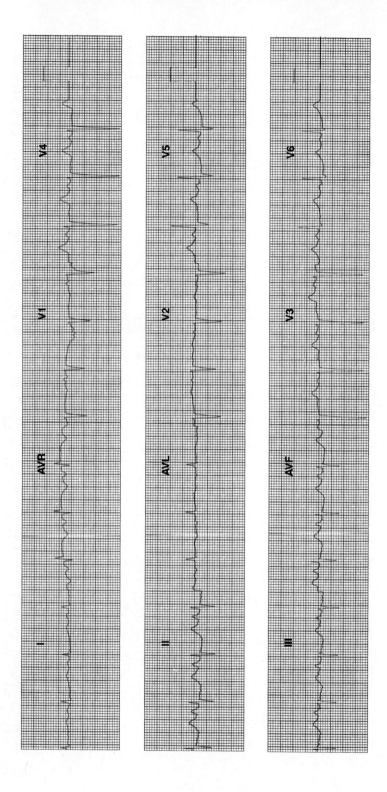

REVIEW ECG 8

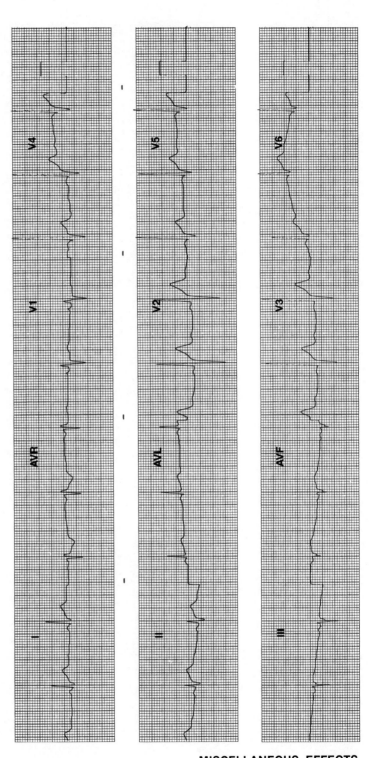

MISCELLANEOUS EFFECTS

REVIEW ECG 9

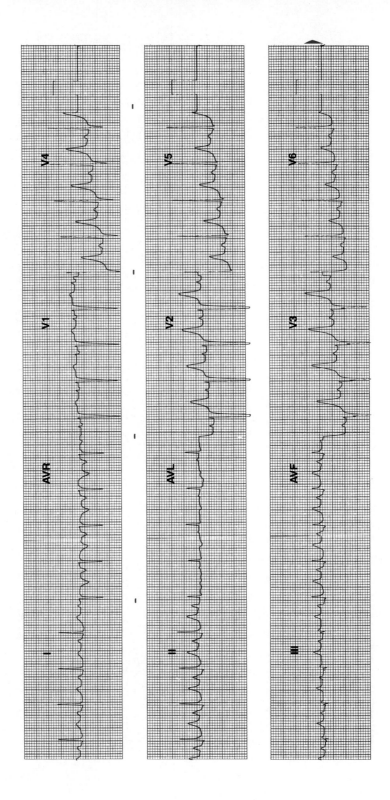

REVIEW ECG 10

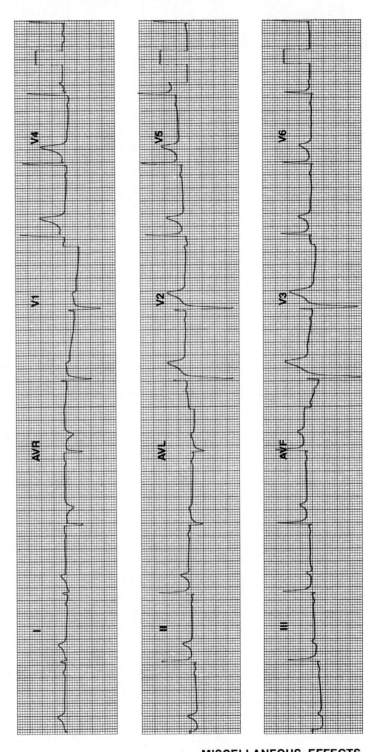

MISCELLANEOUS EFFECTS

REVIEW ECG ANSWERS

1. Sinus tachycardia at 107 per minute with left atrial enlargement and hypercalcemia
2. Sinus bradycardia at 55 per minute with hypokalemia
3. Sinus rhythm at 70 per minute with lateral T wave abnormalities and hypocalcemia
4. Sinus rhythm at 66 per minute with digitalis effect
5. Sinus rhythm at 97 per minute with hyperkalemia and hypocalcemia
6. Sinus rhythm at 62 per minute with first degree AV block, left atrial enlargement, right bundle branch block, and quinidine effect
7. Sinus rhythm at 81 per minute with biatrial enlargement, left anterior hemiblock, possible old anteroseptal infarction, and hypocalcemia
8. Sinus rhythm at 61 per minute with pericarditis versus early repolarization
9. Sinus tachycardia at 107 per minute with biatrial enlargement and hyperkalemia
10. Sinus bradycardia at 54 per minute with probable early repolarization versus pericarditis

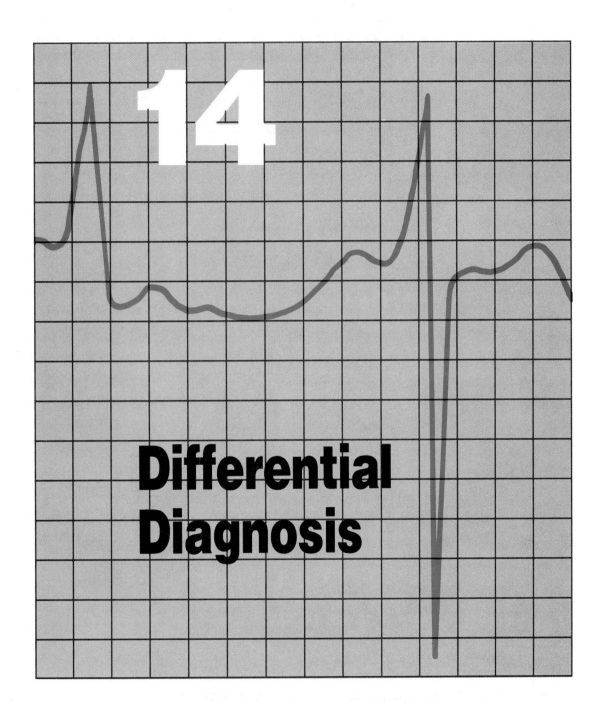

14

Differential Diagnosis

INTERPRETATION METHOD

You should be knowledgeable concerning the criteria for ECG interpretation at this time. At the end of each chapter you've had a chance to become proficient with each new concept learned. Now is the time to establish an easy and organized method for interpreting ECGs using all the criteria in the previous chapters.

1. First the PR and QRS widths are calculated. If the PR interval is greater than .20 second, first degree AV block is present. If the QRS width is greater than .11 second, a bundle branch block is diagnosed. With a diagnosis of bundle branch block, it is necessary to distinguish whether a left or right bundle branch block is occurring. Examine the QRS complexes in lead V_1. A predominantly positive QRS in V_1 with a wide S wave in lead I indicates a right bundle branch block. A predominantly negative QRS in lead V_1 with loss of septal Q waves in the left heart leads illustrates left bundle branch block. It is important to make the correct distinction to make further correct interpretations.

2. The heart rate and rhythm are determined, and the QRS axis of the heart is calculated.

3. Next, atrial enlargements are sought, checking both V_1 for left atrial enlargement and lead II for right atrial enlargement.

4. The ECG is scanned for left and right ventricular hypertrophy. If a left bundle branch block, which indicates abnormal depolarization of the left ventricle, was determined, don't check for other abnormalities of the left ventricle such as left ventricular hypertrophy. And conversely, if right bundle branch block was diagnosed in your initial observations, don't check for right ventricular hypertrophy.

    A right axis is one of the criteria necessary for a diagnosis of right ventricular hypertrophy. If a right axis is not present, as determined during your initial calculations, do not investigate further for right ventricular hypertrophy.

5. Intraventricular conduction disturbances are the next abnormality to scrutinize the ECG for. Using the QRS axis that you calculated earlier, if it is the normal range then both left anterior and left posterior hemiblock can be ruled out. Left anterior hemiblock requires a left axis of −40° or greater, and left posterior hemiblock requires a right axis of +120° or greater. We use the diagnosis of hemiblock when either an abnormal left or right axis is present and there is no other explanation for the abnormal axes.

6. The next step is to determine if a myocardial infarction is present. The ECG is scanned for significant Q waves in all ECG leads except lead aVR. If a left bundle branch block has been previously determined, myocardial infarctions cannot be accurately diagnosed.

   The leads are also inspected for abnormal ST segments and T waves signifying possible ischemia.

7. Lastly, the ECG is examined for miscellaneous effects. The ECG interpretation is then complete.

The most important concept in ECG interpretation is understanding that a single ECG tracing without a clinical history or previous ECGs or both is only one of the many tools for a complete patient evaluation. An ECG alone is often not conclusive of a diagnosis. There are no definites in ECG interpretation, and criteria rules are made to be broken. These rules are only a guide to help you begin honing your interpretive skills. But the guidelines are here to help in making an accurate as possible ECG interpretation while only evaluating a single ECG tracing with no accompanying patient history.

On the following pages, five ECGs with their interpretive readings illustrate this rapid and easy method of ECG interpretation.

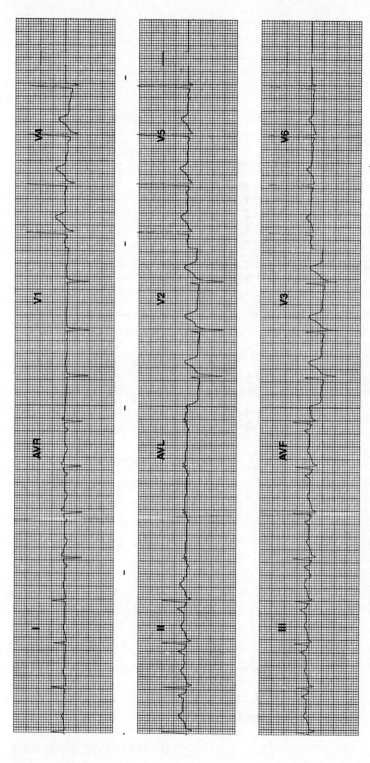

PR and QRS intervals are normal. There is a sinus rhythm at 84 per minute. The QRS axis is normal at +60°. Checking lead V$_1$, left atrial enlargement is not present. Lead II demonstrates right atrial enlargement. Left ventricular hypertrophy criteria are not met, and because there is no right axis, we will not search for right ventricular hypertrophy. Because the axis is normal, neither left anterior hemiblock nor left posterior hemiblock is diagnosed. No significant Q waves of infarction are seen, and the ST-T waves are normal.

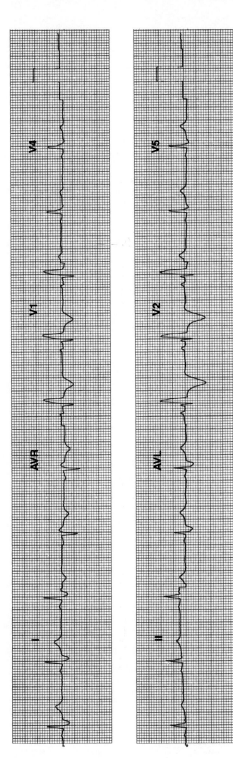

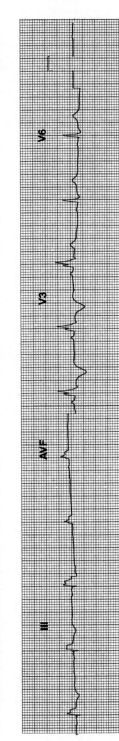

The PR interval is normal, but the QRS interval is wide. Because the QRS complexes are wide and predominantly positive in V$_1$, with a wide S wave in lead I, right bundle branch block is diagnosed. There is sinus rhythm at 60 per minute. The QRS axis is normal at +60°. Left atrial enlargement and right atrial enlargement are not evident. The voltage criteria for left ventricular hypertrophy are not met, and there is no right axis for right ventricular hypertrophy so neither abnormality is diagnosed. Left anterior hemiblock and left posterior hemiblock are not present because the axis is normal. No significant Q waves of infarction are seen, and the only ST-T abnormalities present are the repolarization changes associated with right bundle branch block.

DIFFERENTIAL DIAGNOSIS

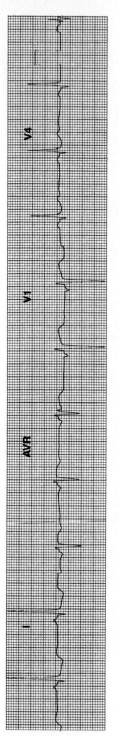

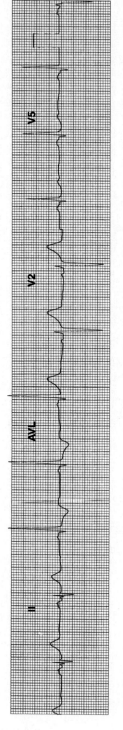

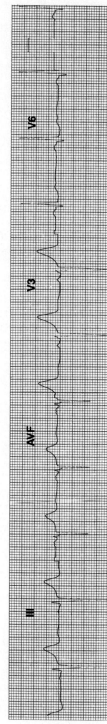

PR and QRS intervals are normal. There is sinus bradycardia at 58 per minute. The QRS axis is left at −30°. Lead V₁ demonstrates the criterion for left atrial enlargement. The criterion for right atrial enlargement is not present. The voltage criteria for left ventricular hypertrophy are met. The axis is not right so right ventricular hypertrophy will not be scanned for. The axis is not far enough left to diagnose left anterior hemiblock. No significant Q waves of infarction are apparent, and the only ST-T abnormalities present are those associated with left ventricular hypertrophy.

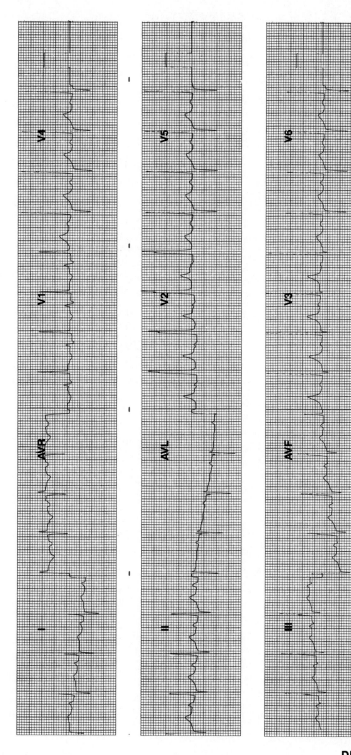

PR and QRS intervals are normal. Sinus rhythm is present at 96 per minute. The QRS axis is right at +105°. V₁ depicts the criterion for left atrial enlargement. The criterion for right atrial enlargement is not met nor are the voltage criteria for left ventricular hypertrophy. Since the axis is right we will look for the voltage criteria of right ventricular hypertrophy and discover that they are met. The axis is right, but that is accounted for by the presence of right ventricular hypertrophy so left posterior hemiblock is not diagnosed. No significant Q waves of infarction are present, and no ST-T abnormalities are seen.

DIFFERENTIAL DIAGNOSIS

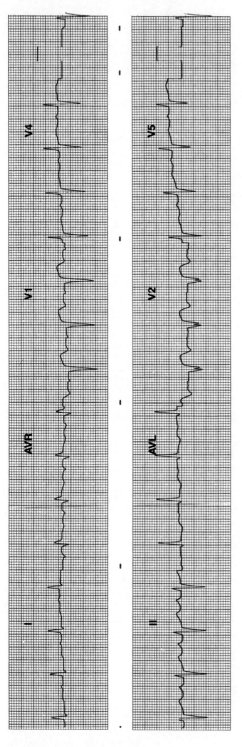

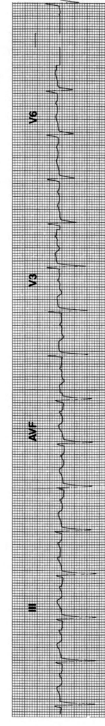

The PR interval is long so first degree AV block is diagnosed. The QRS interval is normal. Sinus rhythm is present at 88 per minute. The QRS axis is left at $-60°$. The criteria for left atrial enlargement and right atrial enlargement are not met. The voltage criteria for left ventricular hypertrophy are not present and because the axis is left, we do not look for right ventricular hypertrophy. The QRS axis is far enough left and no inferior infarction is present so that left anterior hemiblock can be diagnosed. There are significant Q waves in V_1 and V_2 to diagnose an anteroseptal infarction, age indeterminate. Lateral ST-T abnormalities are present.

DIFFERENTIAL DIAGNOSIS

Let's discuss the common problems of differential diagnosis in ECG interpretation in the order in which we investigate for them.

Left and Right Atrial Enlargement. These rarely give any difficulty in diagnosis—either the voltage criteria are met or not. There is no chance of confusing either of these two abnormalities with anything else.

Left Ventricular Hypertrophy. This diagnosis is fairly straightforward. The voltage criteria are usually accompanied by repolarization changes in the left heart leads. One must be careful not to read these repolarization changes in the form of ST-T abnormalities as ischemic changes, but to remember that they are often found with left ventricular hypertrophy. And conversely, be sure not to overlook ischemic changes that can occur along with the repolarization changes. Inverted T waves and ST abnormalities in the inferior leads would not be indicative of repolarization changes of left ventricular hypertrophy. But deeply inverted T waves in the left heart leads, especially if they are symmetrical, even with the diagnosis of left ventricular hypertrophy, would be highly suggestive of accompanying ischemia changes.

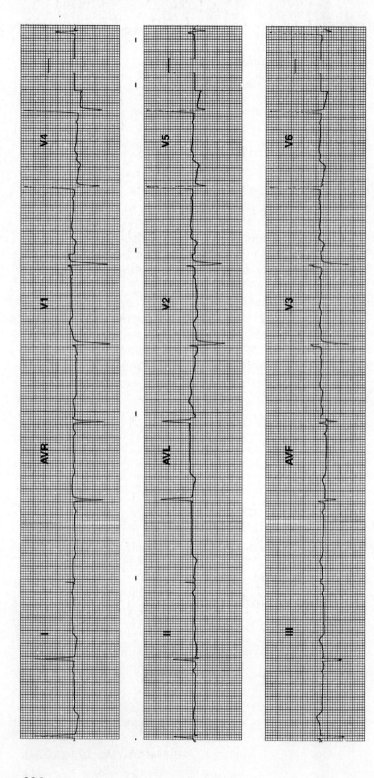

The PR and QRS intervals are normal. There is sinus bradycardia at 49 per minute. The QRS axis is normal. Neither left atrial enlargement nor right atrial enlargement is present. The voltage criteria for left ventricular hypertrophy are met, and there are accompanying repolarization changes in the left heart leads. These are not ischemic changes, but rather the expected ST-T changes of left ventricular hypertrophy. The axis is normal so we don't look for right ventricular hypertrophy. No hemiblocks are diagnosed because the axis is normal. No significant Q waves of infarction are seen.

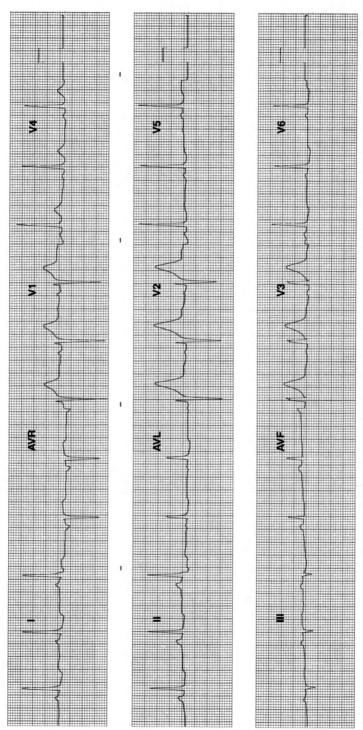

The PR and QRS intervals are normal. There is sinus rhythm at 66 per minute. The QRS axis is normal. Neither left atrial enlargement nor right atrial enlargement is present. The voltage criteria for left ventricular hypertrophy are met, and there are accompanying repolarization changes in the left heart leads. These are not ischemic changes but simply the expected ST-T abnormalities of left ventricular hypertrophy. The axis is normal so we do not look for right ventricular hypertrophy. No hemiblocks are present. No significant Q waves of infarction are seen.

DIFFERENTIAL DIAGNOSIS

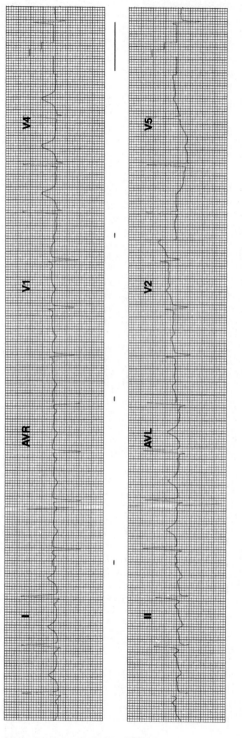

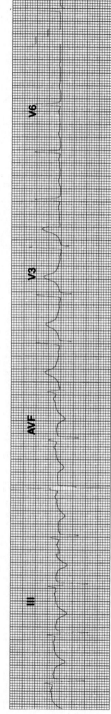

The PR and QRS intervals are normal. There is sinus rhythm at 80 per minute. The QRS axis is slightly leftward. Neither left atrial enlargement nor right atrial enlargement is present. Note that the chest leads are at half standard. The voltage criteria for left ventricular hypertrophy are met, and there are no accompanying repolarization changes in the left heart leads. The axis is not right so right ventricular hypertrophy is not searched for. No hemiblocks are present. There are no significant Q waves of infarction. There are ST-T abnormalities in leads II, III, and aVF. These abnormalities do not represent repolarization changes of left ventricular hypertrophy but rather inferior ischemia.

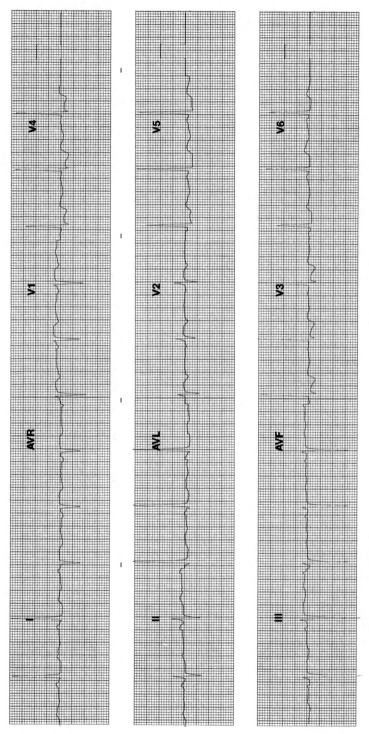

The PR and QRS intervals are normal. Sinus rhythm is present at 69 per minute. The QRS axis is left at −40. Left atrial enlargement and right atrial enlargement are absent. The axis is left at −40 degrees and with the small Q wave in lead I, left anterior hemiblock can be diagnosed. The voltage criteria for left ventricular hypertrophy are met. Repolarization changes of left ventricular hypertrophy are present along with the ST-T changes of ischemia. Right ventricular hypertrophy is not looked for because the QRS axis is normal. No significant Q waves of infarction are apparent.

DIFFERENTIAL DIAGNOSIS

Right Ventricular Hypertrophy. Making a distinction between right ventricular hypertrophy and left posterior hemiblock can often be confusing and at times impossible. Right ventricular hypertrophy requires a right axis plus voltage criteria of an R wave equal or greater than the S wave in lead V_1 or an R wave in V_1 plus the S wave in V_6 equal or greater than 11 mm. Left posterior hemiblock is simply an axis of $+120°$ or greater, a small Q wave in lead III, and no evidence of right ventricular hypertrophy. If you follow the interpretive steps outlined earlier in the chapter, confusion will be kept to a minimum. Don't jump to conclusions during your interpretative process as soon as you see a right axis of $+120°$ or greater and immediately diagnose left posterior hemiblock. Following the steps, you should investigate for right ventricular hypertrophy first. If it is present, then the right axis is explained by the hypertrophy diagnosis.

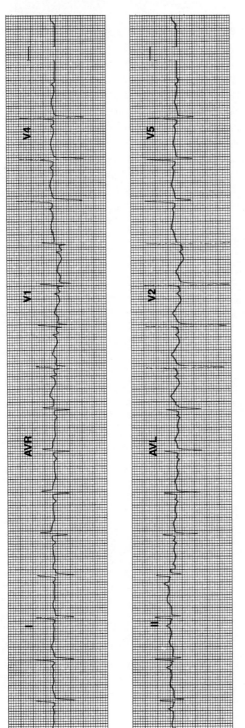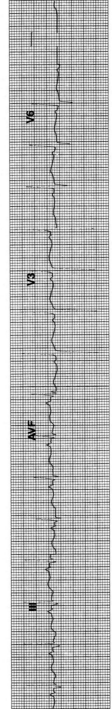

The PR and QRS intervals are normal. There is sinus rhythm at 93 per minute. The QRS axis is right at +120°. Left atrial enlargement and right atrial enlargement are not present. Left ventricular hypertrophy is not present. A right axis is present, and the voltage criteria for right ventricular hypertrophy are met. Although the criteria for left posterior hemiblock are present, right ventricular hypertrophy has been diagnosed and is the reason to investigate first for right ventricular hypertrophy. That is the reason for the right axis. No evidence of infarction is present.

DIFFERENTIAL DIAGNOSIS

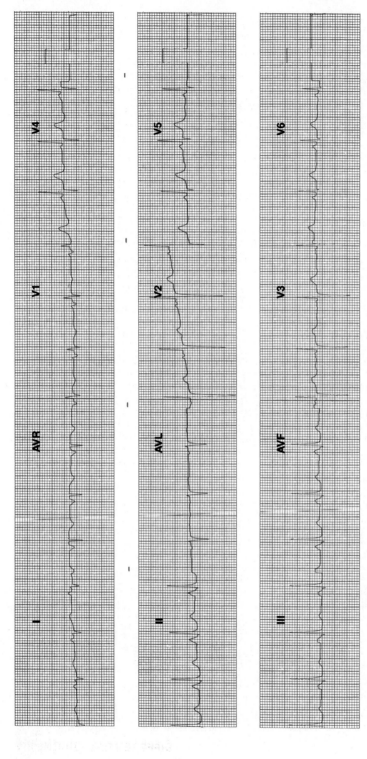

The PR and QRS intervals are normal. Sinus rhythm at 79 per minute is present. The QRS axis is right at +120°. Left atrial enlargement and right atrial enlargement are both diagnosed. Left ventricular hypertrophy is not present. A right axis is present, and the voltage criteria for right ventricular hypertrophy are met. Right ventricular hypertrophy is diagnosed, and the explanation for the right axis is evident, ruling out the diagnosis of left posterior hemiblock. No evidence of infarction is seen.

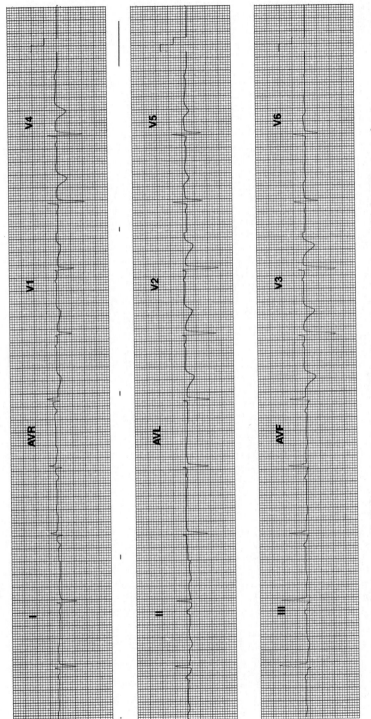

The PR and QRS intervals are normal. There is sinus bradycardia at 58 per minute. The QRS axis is +120°. Left atrial enlargement and right atrial enlargement are absent. Left ventricular hypertrophy criteria are not met. Although a right axis is present, the voltage criteria for right ventricular hypertrophy are not met. The criteria for left posterior hemiblock are present. No significant Q waves of infarction are present, but anterolateral ischemia is diagnosed.

DIFFERENTIAL DIAGNOSIS

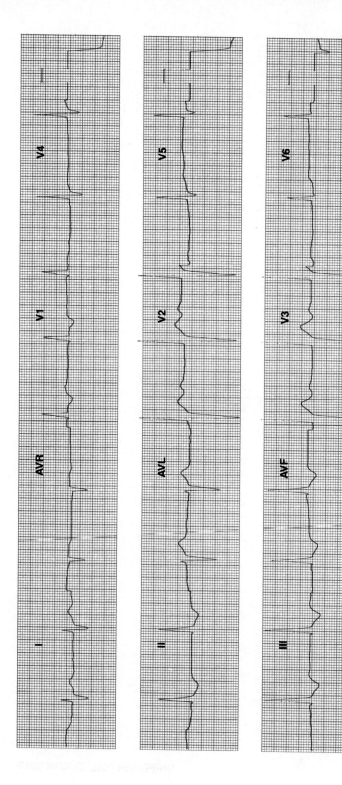

Atrial fibrillation is present so there is no PR interval. The QRS is widened, predominantly positive in V_1, and a wide S wave is seen in lead I, indicating right bundle branch block. The QRS axis is +120°. Neither left atrial enlargement nor right atrial enlargement is present. Left ventricular hypertrophy is not present, and right ventricular hypertrophy is not diagnosed in the presence of right bundle branch block. With an axis of +120° and a small Q wave in lead III, a diagnosis of left posterior hemiblock is made. No significant Q waves of infarction are present.

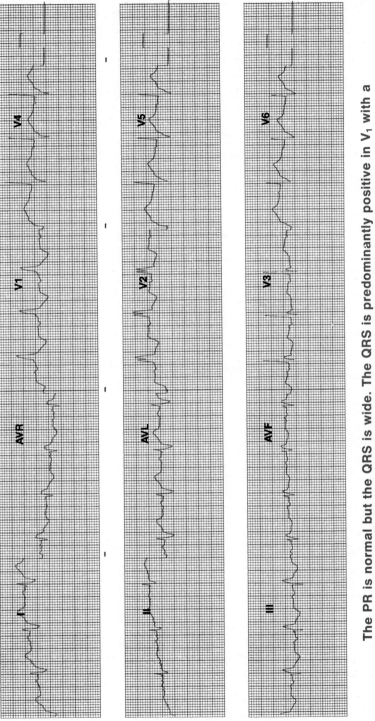

The PR is normal but the QRS is wide. The QRS is predominantly positive in V$_1$ with a wide S wave in lead I making the diagnosis of right bundle branch block correct. There is sinus rhythm at 87 per minute. The QRS axis is +120°. Left atrial enlargement and right atrial enlargement are absent. Left ventricular hypertrophy is not present, and right ventricular hypertrophy is not diagnosed in the presence of right bundle branch block. With an axis of +120° and a small Q wave in lead III, left posterior hemiblock is diagnosed. No significant Q waves of infarction are seen.

DIFFERENTIAL DIAGNOSIS

Right Bundle Branch Block. This is not confused with any other diagnosis, but it can mask other abnormalities. Repolarization changes accompanying right bundle branch block may mask the diagnosis of ischemia. The repolarization changes of right bundle branch block are found in the right heart leads. Be sure not to label ST-T abnormalities in the left heart leads as repolarization changes when they may actually be ischemic or nondiagnostic ST-T abnormalities.

If you scan the ECG too quickly when right bundle branch block is present, you might not see significant Q waves of infarction in the widened QRS complexes. Check each QRS complex carefully for all abnormalities.

Incomplete right bundle branch block is similar to that of right bundle branch block except the QRS complex is slightly under .12 second.

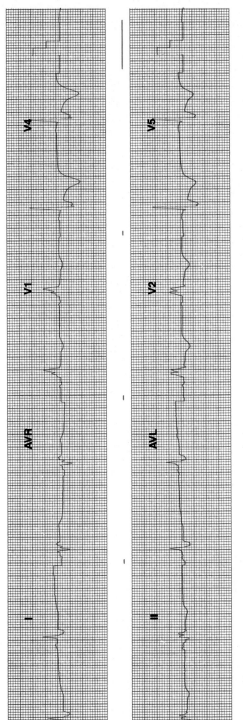
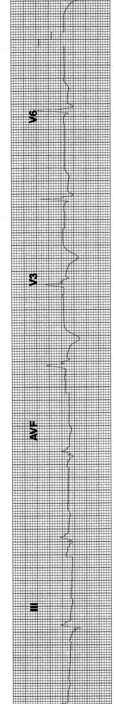

The PR is normal but the QRS is wide. Right bundle branch block is present with a predominantly positive QRS in V_1 and a wide S wave in lead I. There is sinus bradycardia at 45 per minute. The QRS axis is 0°. Left atrial enlargement and right atrial enlargement are not present. Left ventricular hypertrophy is not present, and right ventricular hypertrophy is not diagnosed in the presence of right bundle branch block. The axis is normal so hemiblocks are absent. Significant Q waves are seen in leads II, III, and aVF, indicating an inferior infarction, age indeterminate. The ST-T abnormalities are not repolarization changes of right bundle branch block but suggest anterolateral ischemia.

DIFFERENTIAL DIAGNOSIS

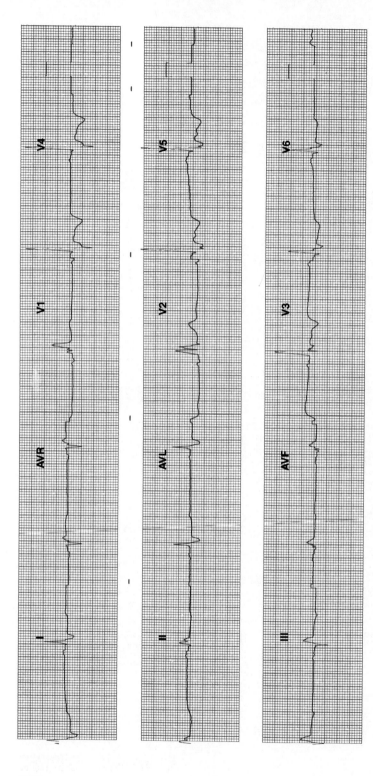

The PR is normal, and the QRS is wide and represents right bundle branch block. Sinus bradycardia at 39 per minute is present. The QRS axis is 0°. Neither left atrial enlargement nor right atrial enlargement is present. Left ventricular hypertrophy and right ventricular hypertrophy are diagnosed. No hemiblocks are absent. No hemiblocks are present and are infarction are not in evidence. Anterolateral ST-T abnormalities are present and are not indicative of the repolarization changes of right bundle branch block because they are occurring in the left heart leads.

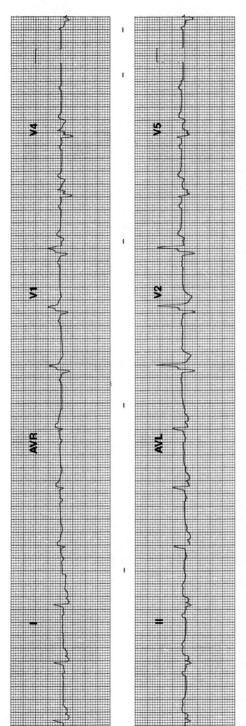

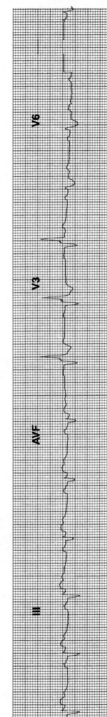

The PR is normal. The QRS is wide and represents right bundle branch block. There is sinus rhythm at 66 per minute. The QRS axis is −15°. Left atrial enlargement and right atrial enlargement are not present. Left ventricular hypertrophy and right ventricular hypertrophy are absent. No hemiblocks are diagnosed. Do not miss the Q waves of infarction in both the anterior and inferior leads. The anterior infarction is of an age indeterminate; the inferior infarction may be acute. There are ST-T abnormalities in the lateral leads. Do not assume that these ST-T abnormalities are part of the repolarization changes of right bundle branch block. The repolarization changes of right bundle branch block are in the right heart leads only.

DIFFERENTIAL DIAGNOSIS

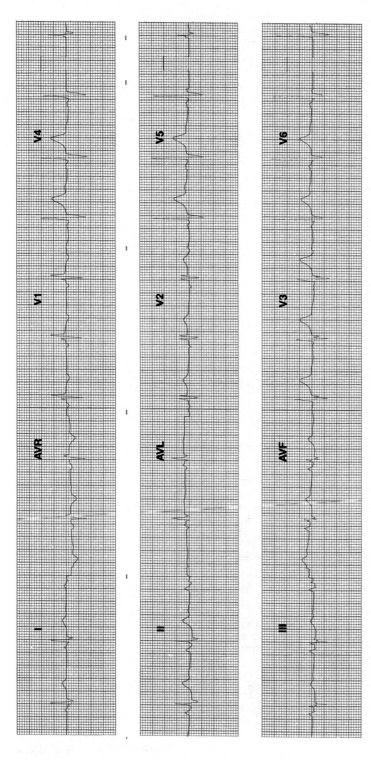

The PR and QRS intervals are of normal duration. There is sinus rhythm at 64 per minute. The QRS axis is +30°. Left atrial enlargement and right atrial enlargement are not present. Left ventricular hypertrophy and right ventricular hypertrophy are absent. Although the QRS axis is not widened, there is an RsR′ pattern in V_1, and lead I displays a slightly widened S wave indicating an incomplete right bundle branch block. Neither left anterior hemiblock nor left posterior hemiblock is present. No significant Q waves are present.

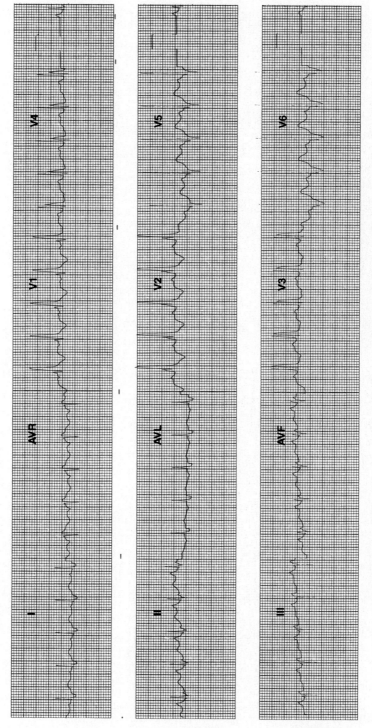

The PR and QRS intervals are normal. There is sinus rhythm at 118 per minute. The QRS axis is 0°. Left atrial enlargement and right atrial enlargement are not present. Left ventricular hypertrophy and right ventricular hypertrophy are absent. The QRS is almost .12 second in duration and has a predominantly positive QRS in V_1, and a widened S wave in lead I, indicating incomplete right bundle branch block. No hemiblocks are present, and there are no significant Q waves of infarction.

DIFFERENTIAL DIAGNOSIS

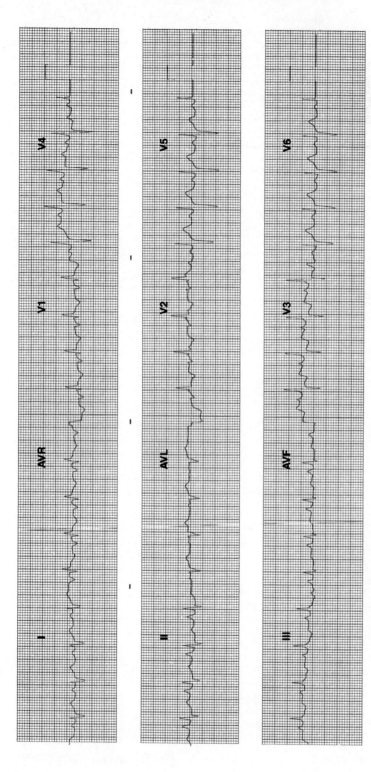

The PR and QRS intervals are normal. There is sinus tachycardia at 106 per minute. The QRS axis is +120°. Biatrial enlargement is diagnosed. Left ventricular hypertrophy is not present. The QRS is almost .12 second wide and has a predominantly positive QRS in V_1 and a widened S wave in lead I, indicating incomplete right bundle branch block. A right axis and an R wave as large as the S wave in lead V_1 indicate a probable right ventricular hypertrophy in the presence of incomplete right bundle branch block. No hemiblocks are diagnosed, and no significant Q waves are seen.

Left Bundle Branch Block. This intraventricular conduction disturbance isn't confused with any other diagnosis but often masks other abnormalities.

Never diagnose infarction in the presence of left bundle branch block. If you follow the order of interpretation that we've been using, you'll discover a left bundle branch block before you begin to look for significant Q waves of infarction and you won't be fooled.

The repolarization changes of this intraventricular conduction disturbance can also mimic ischemic ST-T changes in the left heart leads.

A widened QRS complex, resembling left bundle branch block, but without the loss of septal Q waves is referred to as a nonspecific intraventricular conduction disturbance. When this is correctly identified, left ventricular hypertrophy and infarction can be diagnosed accurately.

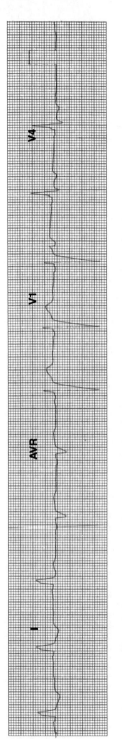

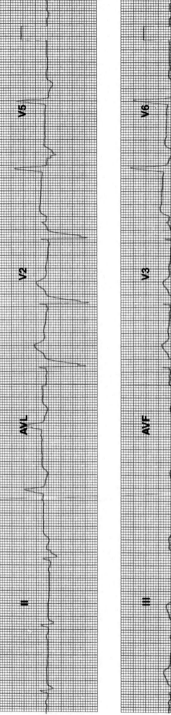

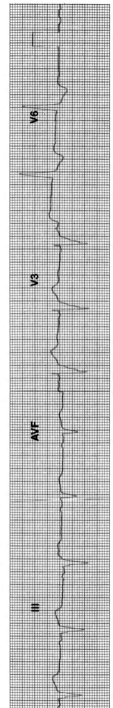

The PR interval is normal. The QRS is widened, the QRS is predominantly negative in lead V_1, and a loss of septal Q waves indicates left bundle branch block. There is sinus bradycardia at 59 per minute. The QRS axis is −30°. Left atrial enlargement and right atrial enlargement are not present. Left ventricular hypertrophy is not diagnosed in the presence of left bundle branch block, and right ventricular hypertrophy is not indicated. Because left bundle branch block is present, neither the left anterior nor posterior fascicle is conducting electrical impulses. We do not use the term hemiblock when left bundle branch block is diagnosed. Do not attempt to diagnose infarction in the presence of left bundle branch block. The evident ST-T changes represent those accompanying left bundle branch block and not those of ischemia.

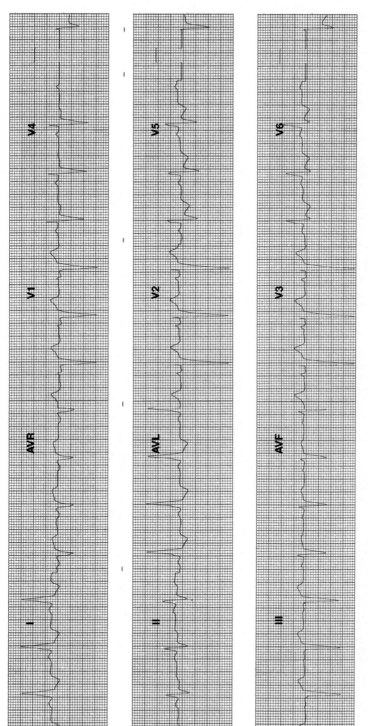

The PR interval is normal. The QRS is widened and represents left bundle branch block. There is sinus rhythm at 81 per minute. The QRS axis is −30°. Left atrial enlargement is present; right atrial enlargement is not. Left ventricular hypertrophy is not diagnosed in the presence of left bundle branch block. Right ventricular hypertrophy is not indicated. Because of left bundle branch block, hemiblocks are not diagnosed. No attempt at infarction diagnosis is made in the presence of left bundle branch block. The ST-T abnormalities represent the repolarization changes of left bundle branch block.

DIFFERENTIAL DIAGNOSIS

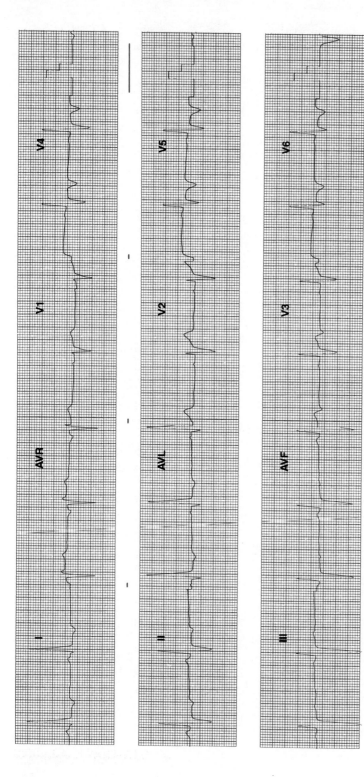

The PR interval is normal. The QRS is widened, predominantly negative in lead V_1, but septal Q waves are present, indicating a nonspecific intraventricular conduction disturbance. With this diagnosis, both left ventricular hypertrophy and infarction can be diagnosed, and left ventricular hypertrophy is present. There is sinus bradycardia at 50 per minute. The QRS axis is −30. Neither left anterior hemiblock nor left posterior hemiblock is present. No significant Q waves of infarction are present.

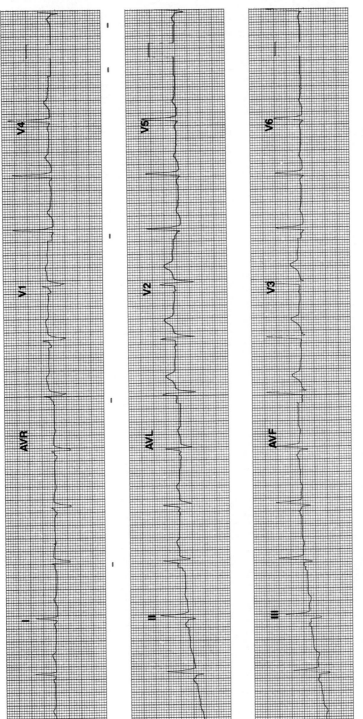

The PR interval is normal. The QRS is widened, predominantly negative in lead V_1, but septal Q waves are present indicating a nonspecific intraventricular conduction disturbance. Sinus rhythm is present at 70 per minute. The QRS axis is +60°. Left atrial enlargement is present. Neither left ventricular hypertrophy nor right ventricular hypertrophy is present. Left anterior hemiblock and left posterior hemiblock are absent. The significant Q waves in leads II, III, and aVF, accompanied by inverted T waves, signify an inferior infarction, age indeterminate.

DIFFERENTIAL DIAGNOSIS

Left Anterior Hemiblock. This abnormality is diagnosed predominantly by its left axis with a small Q wave in lead I. You should be sure that a left axis of −40°, necessary for left anterior hemiblock, is not caused by deep Q waves of an inferior infarction. An acute inferior infarction would probably not be overlooked, but an old infarction without the elevated ST segments or inverted T waves might cause the incorrect diagnosis of left anterior hemiblock.

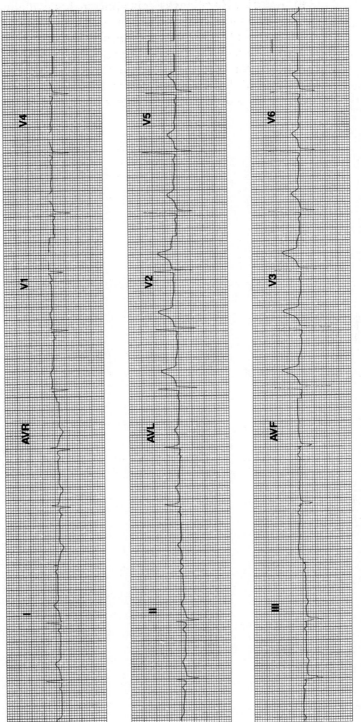

The PR and QRS intervals are normal. Sinus rhythm is present at 66 per minute. The QRS axis is −60°. Left atrial enlargement and right atrial enlargement are absent. Left ventricular hypertrophy and right ventricular hypertrophy are not present. Left anterior hemiblock is diagnosed because the axis is over −40°, there is a small Q wave in lead I, and there is no evidence of an inferior infarction. No significant Q waves are seen.

DIFFERENTIAL DIAGNOSIS

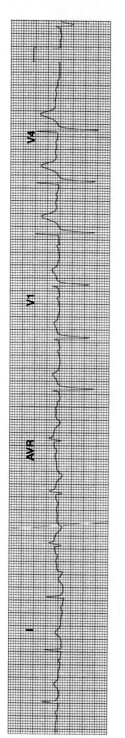

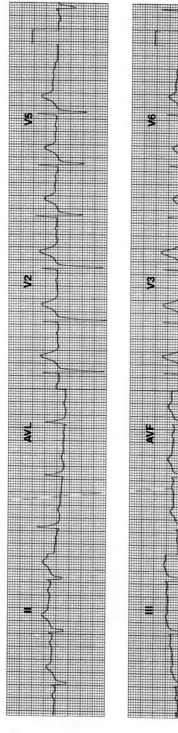

The PR and QRS intervals are normal. There is sinus rhythm at 74 per minute. The QRS axis is −60°. Left atrial enlargement and right atrial enlargement are absent. The criteria for left ventricular hypertrophy and right ventricular hypertrophy are not met. The axis is far left and a small Q wave is present in lead I indicating left anterior hemiblock. Leads II, III, and aVF all have small R waves present rather than QS waves. The diagnosis of inferior Q waves would be incorrect. If you interpret too quickly, a diagnosis of inferior infarction might be incorrectly made. No significant Q waves are seen.

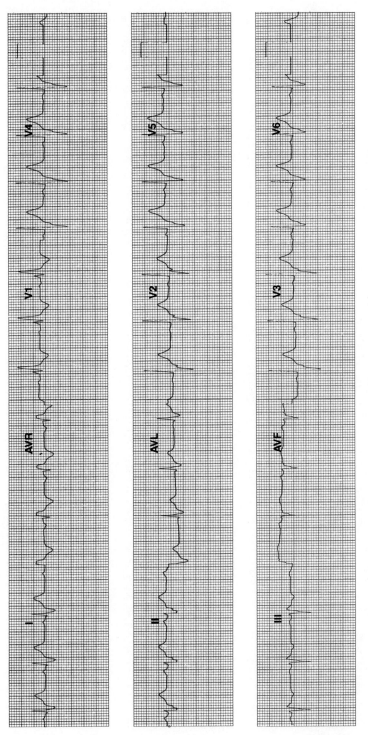

The PR interval is normal. The QRS is wide and indicates right bundle branch block. There is sinus rhythm at 81 per minute. The QRS axis is −60°. Left atrial enlargement and right atrial enlargement are not present. Left ventricular hypertrophy and right ventricular hypertrophy are absent. Because the axis is over −40°, there is a small Q wave in lead I, and there is no evidence of an inferior infarction left anterior hemiblock is diagnosed. A bifascicular block is present—right bundle branch block and left anterior hemiblock. No evidence of infarction is seen.

DIFFERENTIAL DIAGNOSIS

319

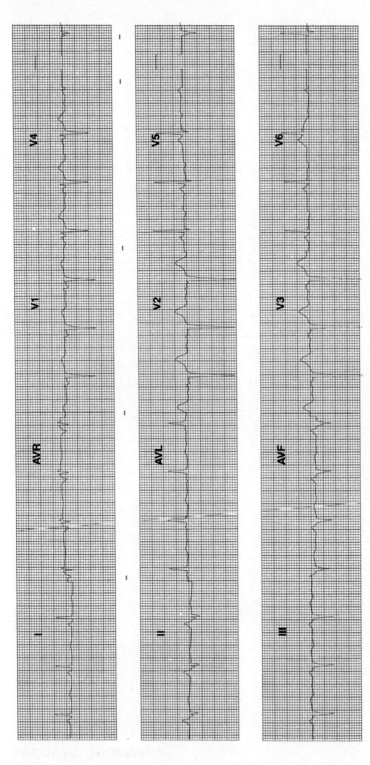

The PR and QRS intervals are normal. There is sinus rhythm at 80 per minute. The QRS axis is −60°. Both left atrial enlargement and right atrial enlargement are diagnosed. Neither left ventricular hypertrophy nor right ventricular hypertrophy is present. The axis is over −40° and there is a small Q wave in lead I, but there is evidence of an old inferior infarction which is causing the left axis by its deep QS waves. Therefore, left anterior hemiblock is not present. An anterior infarction should be considered because of the extremely poor R wave progression.

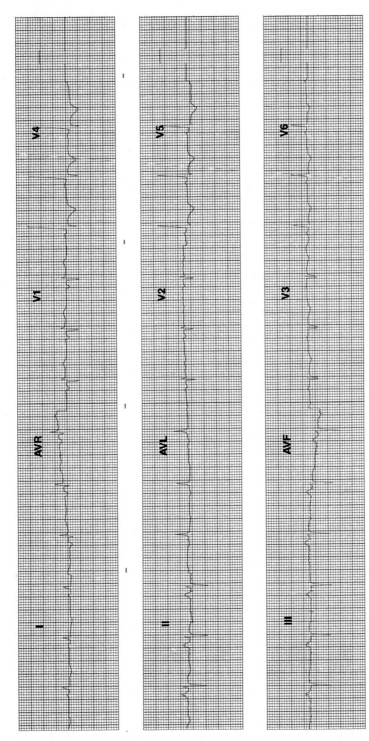

The PR and QRS intervals are normal. Sinus rhythm is present at 76 per minute. The QRS axis is −60°. Both left atrial enlargement and right atrial enlargement are present. Neither left ventricular hypertrophy nor right ventricular hypertrophy is diagnosed. The QRS axis is over −40°, there is no inferior infarction, but there is no Q wave in lead I negating a diagnosis of left anterior hemiblock. Left posterior hemiblock is not present. An anterior infarction, age indeterminate, is diagnosed, and lateral T wave abnormalities are noted—possibly ischemic.

DIFFERENTIAL DIAGNOSIS

Left Posterior Hemiblock. This abnormality is not seen as often as its counterpart, left anterior hemiblock, and is diagnosed predominantly by a right axis of +120° or greater and a small Q wave in lead III. If right ventricular hypertrophy is diagnosed, the right axis is present because of the increased vectors associated with the enlarged right ventricle and not because of left posterior hemiblock. Again, if you religiously follow the method of interpretation outlined for you, you'll have no problem in distinguishing between the two.

Sometimes, a lateral infarction with deep Q waves in leads I and aVL will cause a right axis deviation. If there is a logical reason for the right axis of +120° or greater, such as a lateral infarction or right ventricular hypertrophy, then left posterior hemiblock can be ruled out.

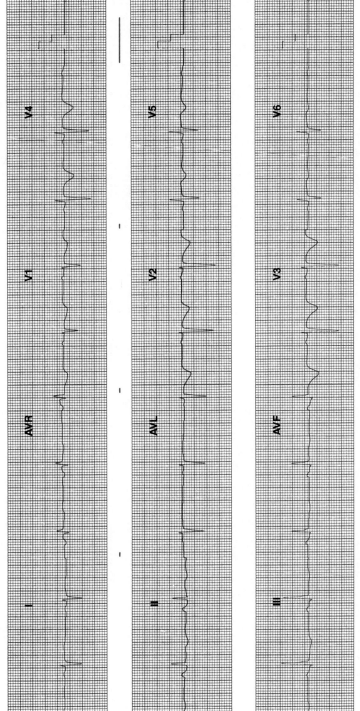

The PR and QRS intervals are normal. There is sinus bradycardia at 58 per minute. The QRS axis is +120°. Neither left atrial enlargement nor right atrial enlargement is present. Left ventricular hypertrophy and right ventricular hypertrophy are absent. The QRS axis is +120°, there is a small Q wave in lead III, and there is no evidence of right ventricular hypertrophy, indicating left posterior hemiblock. No significant Q waves of infarction are seen, but anterolateral ischemia is present.

DIFFERENTIAL DIAGNOSIS

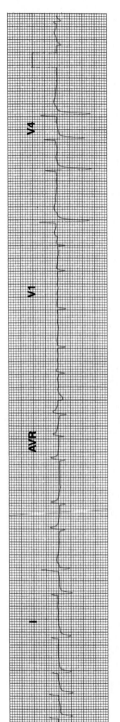
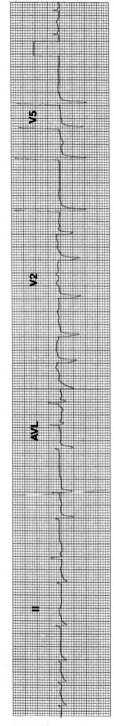
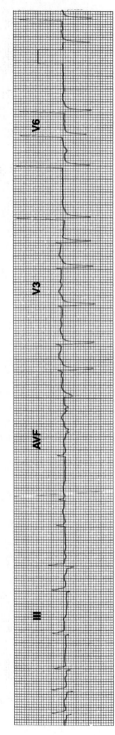

Atrial fibrillation is diagnosed so no PR interval is present. The QRS interval is normal. The QRS axis is +120°. Neither left atrial enlargement nor right atrial enlargement can be diagnosed. Neither left ventricular hypertrophy nor right ventricular hypertrophy is present. Because the axis is +120°, a small Q wave is present in lead III, and there is no evidence of right ventricular hypertrophy, left posterior hemiblock is diagnosed. Poor R wave progression in leads V_1–V_3 suggests an anteroseptal infarct, probably old. Anterolateral ST-T abnormalities are noted.

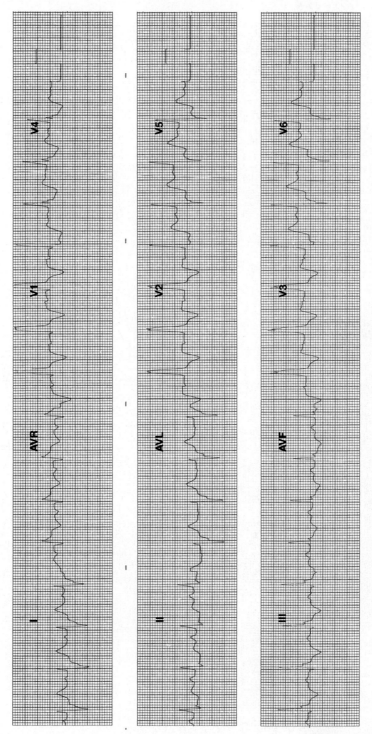

The PR interval is normal, but the QRS interval is wide. Right bundle branch block is present. The QRS axis is +120°. Left atrial enlargement is present. Neither left ventricular hypertrophy nor right ventricular hypertrophy is present. Left posterior hemiblock is diagnosed because of the right axis of +120°, a small Q wave in lead III, and no evidence of right ventricular hypertrophy. No evidence of infarction is seen. ST depression is noted throughout the tracing.

DIFFERENTIAL DIAGNOSIS

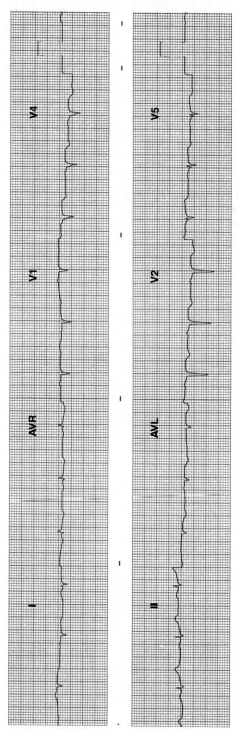

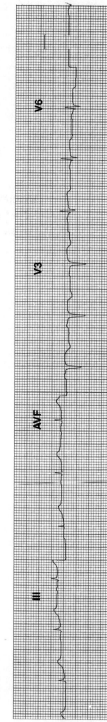

The PR and QRS intervals are normal. Sinus rhythm is present at 75 per minute. The QRS axis is +120°. Neither left atrial enlargement nor right atrial enlargement is seen. Left ventricular hypertrophy and right ventricular hypertrophy are absent. There is a right axis of +120°, there is a small Q wave in lead III, and there is no evidence of right ventricular hypertrophy, all leading one to suspect left posterior hemiblock. But on careful inspection, the right axis is caused by the Q waves of the lateral infarction not left posterior hemiblock. An anterior infarction is also present. Both infarctions are of an indeterminate age.

Infarction. The diagnosis of inferior, lateral, and anterior infarctions is contingent on finding significant Q waves in at least two leads for each infarct location, or in the case of anterior infarctions, poor R wave progression in leads V_1–V_3.

It is common to see small Q waves in the anterior and lateral leads, as these represent septal Q waves and are not considered significant of infarction. Q waves are uncommon in the inferior leads, and although they may not be significant, it is noteworthy to mention their existence.

Q waves in V_1 and V_2 or poor R wave progression may also be due to left ventricular hypertrophy.

Diagnosing a posterior infarction requires tall R waves, often accompanied by tall T waves, in V_1 and V_2. Making the diagnosis in the company of an inferior infarction is easier and more reliable than trying to diagnose a posterior infarction alone. Once an inferior infarction is determined, leads V_1 and V_2 should be checked for tall R waves. ST segments in V_1 and V_2 are often depressed in the case of an acute posterior infarction. These criteria for posterior infarction represent the exact opposite of what we routinely check for in infarction—

Tall R wave instead of deep Q wave
Depressed ST segment instead of elevated ST segment
Tall upright T waves instead of inverted T waves

because the posterior wall has no electrodes directly on it as do all the other infarct locations.

Remember, infarctions should not be diagnosed in the presence of left bundle branch block. The right ventricle depolarizes before the left in left bundle branch block, so any Q waves of infarction would be buried within the QRS complex rather than appearing at the beginning.

Once an infarction has been diagnosed, the age of the infarct must be determined. Elevated ST segments indicate an acute infarct. Inverted T waves imply an infarct of an indeterminate age, possibly recent or older, and an old infarct simply demonstrates a Q wave with no ST-T abnormalities. Making an exact determination of infarction age from an isolated ECG is difficult, and obtaining serial ECGs over a period of days or weeks would be more exact.

DIFFERENTIAL DIAGNOSIS

327

Ischemia is demonstrated by ST depression or T wave inversion. T waves can be normally inverted in leads III, aVR, and V_1. It is often difficult to make the diagnosis of ischemia from an ECG tracing alone. So unless the tracing demonstrates deeply inverted T waves or very deep ST depression, the diagnosis of nondiagnostic ST-T abnormalities is often used. Serial ECGs or clinical correlation is often necessary to confirm the diagnosis of ischemia.

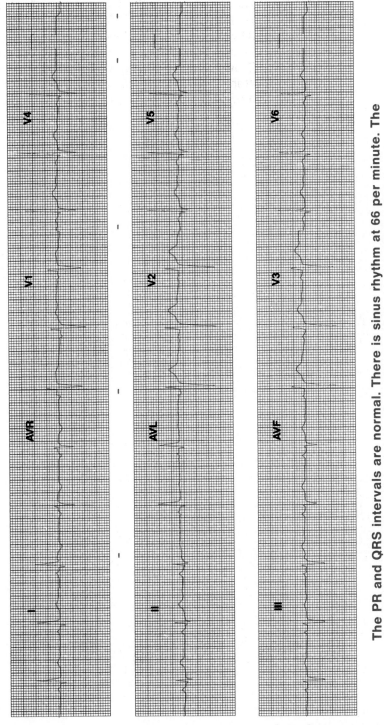

The PR and QRS intervals are normal. There is sinus rhythm at 66 per minute. The QRS axis is −30°. Left atrial enlargement and right atrial enlargement are not present. Left ventricular hypertrophy and right ventricular hypertrophy are not present. No hemiblocks are diagnosed. There are septal Q waves in all the left heart leads—these are not Q waves of infarction.

DIFFERENTIAL DIAGNOSIS

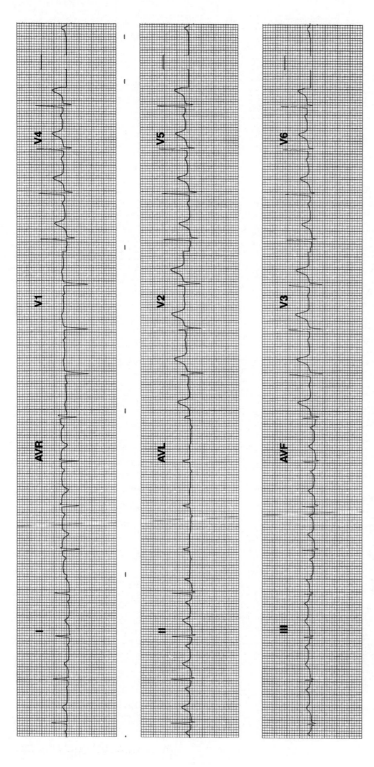

The PR and QRS intervals are normal. There is a sinus rhythm at 87 per minute. The QRS axis is +60°. Neither left atrial enlargement nor right atrial enlargement is present. Left ventricular hypertrophy and right ventricular hypertrophy are not seen. No hemiblocks are diagnosed. One significant Q wave is noted in lead V_1, but two are required for the diagnosis of infarction.

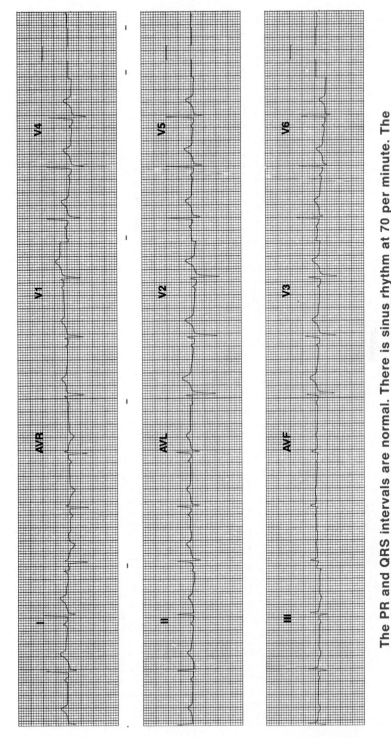

The PR and QRS intervals are normal. There is sinus rhythm at 70 per minute. The QRS axis is 0°. Left atrial enlargement and right atrial enlargement are not present. Left ventricular hypertrophy and right ventricular hypertrophy are not evident. No hemiblocks are present. There is one significant Q wave noted in lead III, but two are needed in each infarct location for the diagnosis of infarction.

DIFFERENTIAL DIAGNOSIS

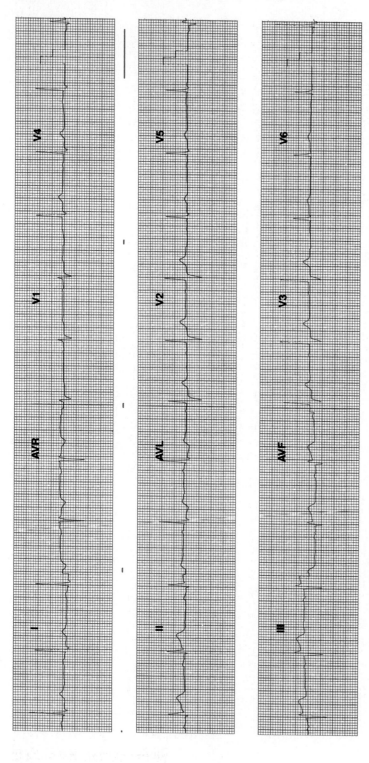

The PR and QRS intervals are normal. There is sinus rhythm at 62 per minute. The QRS axis is 0°. Left atrial enlargement and right atrial enlargement are absent. Neither left ventricular hypertrophy nor right ventricular hypertrophy is diagnosed. No hemiblocks are present. There are significant Q waves in leads III and aVF, indicating an inferior infarction. The ST segments are elevated in the inferior leads, signifying an acute inferior infarction.

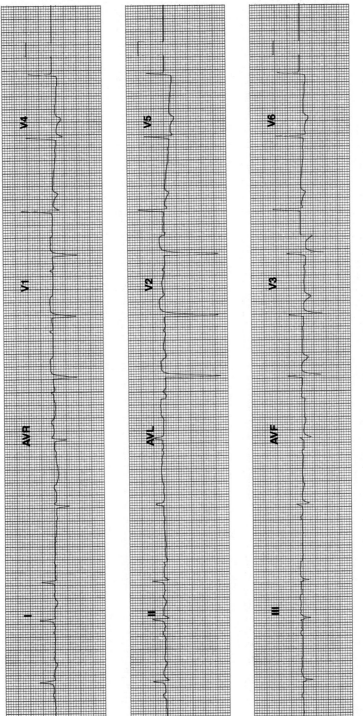

There is first degree AV block. The QRS interval is normal. Sinus rhythm is present at 60 per minute. The QRS axis is 0°. Left atrial enlargement and right atrial enlargement are absent. Left ventricular hypertrophy and right ventricular hypertrophy are not present. No hemiblocks are present. There are significant Q waves in leads V_1 and V_2 accompanied by ST segment elevations and T wave inversion, indicating an acute anteroseptal infarction. There is T wave inversion noted throughout the tracing with questionable significance. One atrial premature contraction is noted.

DIFFERENTIAL DIAGNOSIS

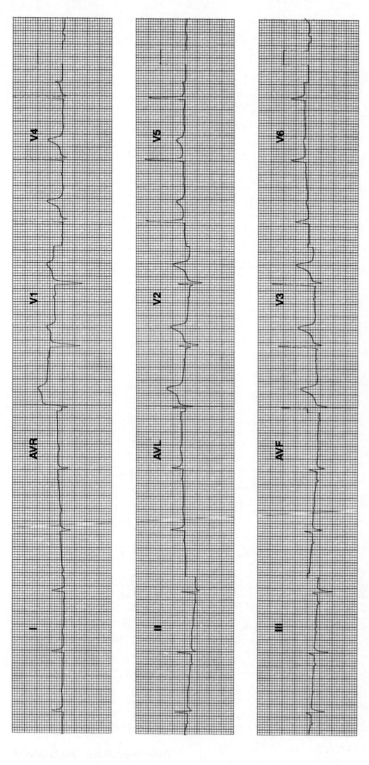

First degree AV block is present. The QRS interval is normal. Sinus rhythm is present at 63 per minute. The QRS axis is 0°. Left atrial enlargement and right atrial enlargement are absent. Neither left ventricular hypertrophy nor right ventricular hypertrophy is present. No hemiblocks are present. There are significant Q waves in leads V_1 and V_2 with no ST-T abnormalities, indicating an old anteroseptal infarction. Inferior ST-T abnormalities are seen.

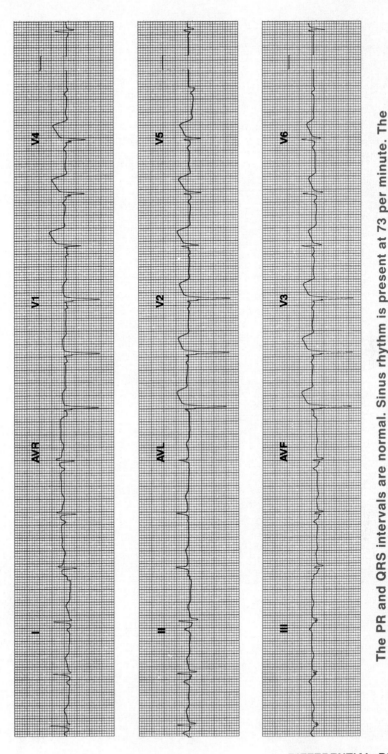

The PR and QRS intervals are normal. Sinus rhythm is present at 73 per minute. The QRS axis is 0°. Right atrial enlargement is present. Left ventricular hypertrophy and right ventricular hypertrophy are absent. There is poor R wave progression across the precordium accompanied by elevated ST segments, indicating an acute anterior infarction. There is a possible inferior infarction, age indeterminate.

DIFFERENTIAL DIAGNOSIS

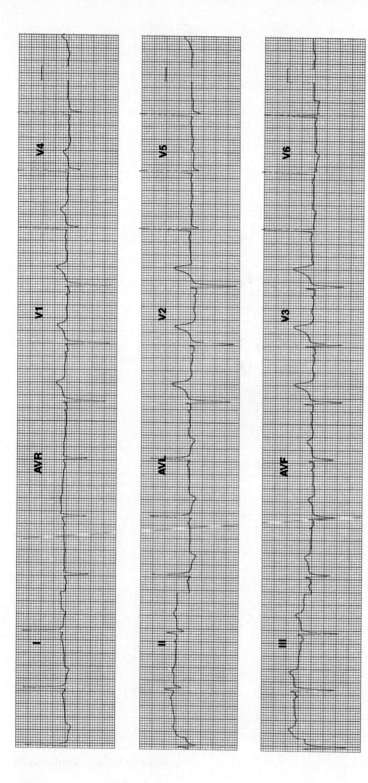

The PR and QRS intervals are normal. Sinus rhythm is present at 67 per minute. The QRS axis is −15°. Neither left atrial enlargement nor right atrial enlargement is seen. Left ventricular hypertrophy is present. No hemiblocks are seen. There is poor R wave progression across the precordium, but this is probably due to the left ventricular hypertrophy rather than an anterior infarction.

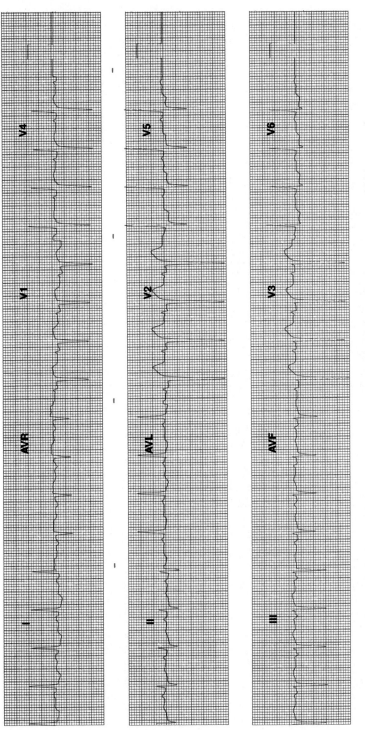

The PR and QRS intervals are normal. Sinus tachycardia is present at 101 per minute. The QRS axis is −30°. Left atrial enlargement and right atrial enlargement are not evident. Left ventricular hypertrophy is present. Hemiblocks are absent. Significant Q waves and poor R wave progression are seen in leads V_1–V_3, but this is probably attributed to the left ventricular hypertrophy. If left ventricular hypertrophy were not diagnosed, an anteroseptal infarction would be suspected.

DIFFERENTIAL DIAGNOSIS

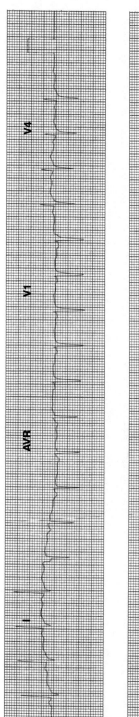
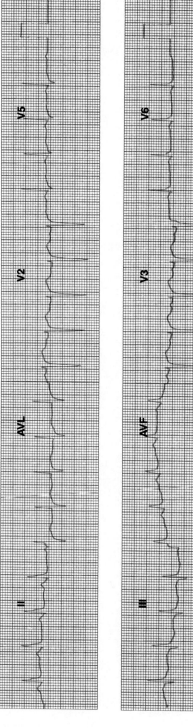

The PR and QRS intervals are normal. Sinus tachycardia is present at 109 per minute. The QRS axis is 0°. No enlargements or hypertrophies are present. Hemiblocks are absent. There are Q waves in the inferior leads, but only lead III has a significant Q wave. There is poor R wave progression across the precordium indicating an old anterior infarction. There are nonspecific ST-T abnormalities throughout the tracing.

338

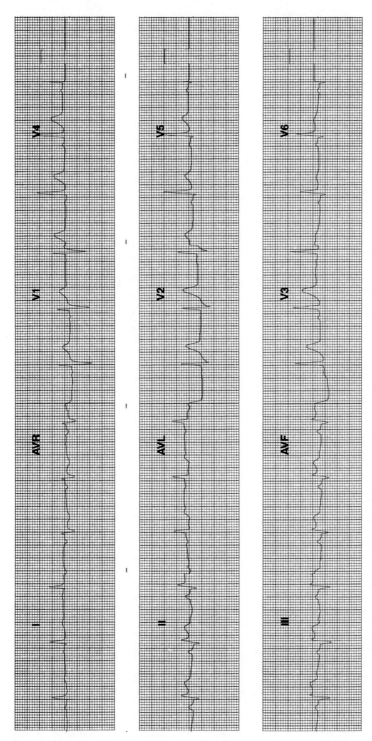

The PR and QRS intervals are normal. There is sinus rhythm at 69 per minute. The QRS axis is 0°. Left atrial enlargement and right atrial enlargement are absent. Neither left ventricular hypertrophy nor right ventricular hypertrophy is present. No hemiblocks are diagnosed. Significant Q waves are seen in leads II, III, and aVF with elevated ST segments, signifying an acute inferior infarction. There are also tall R waves in leads V_1 and V_2, accompanied by tall T waves and ST depression, indicating an acute posterior infarct.

DIFFERENTIAL DIAGNOSIS

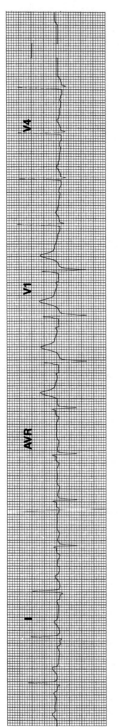

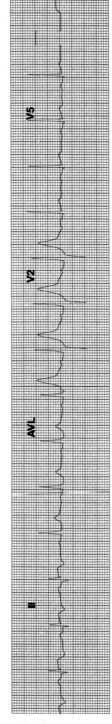

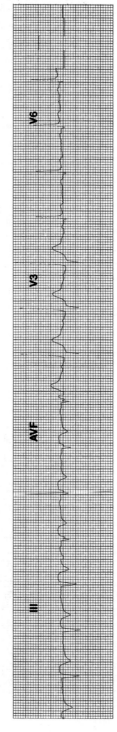

The PR and QRS intervals are normal. There is sinus rhythm at 84 per minute. The QRS axis is 0°. Neither left atrial enlargement nor right atrial enlargement is evident. Left ventricular hypertrophy and right ventricular hypertrophy are not present. No hemiblocks are seen. There are significant Q waves in the inferior leads accompanied by elevated ST segments and inverted T waves, indicating this is probably an acute or at least a recent infarction. There are also tall R waves and T waves in leads V$_1$ and V$_2$ with ST segment depression, allowing a diagnosis of an acute posterior infarction.

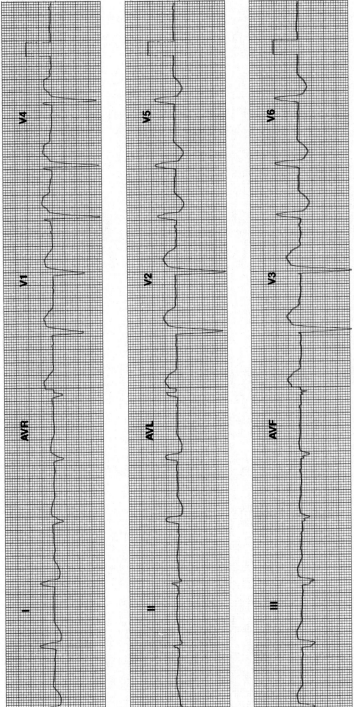

The PR is normal. The QRS interval is wide and represents left bundle branch block. Left atrial enlargement and right atrial enlargement are absent. Neither left ventricular hypertrophy nor right ventricular hypertrophy is present. Hemiblocks are not scanned for because of left bundle branch block. Although it appears that anterior and inferior infarctions are present, infarctions are not diagnosed in the presence of left bundle branch block.

DIFFERENTIAL DIAGNOSIS

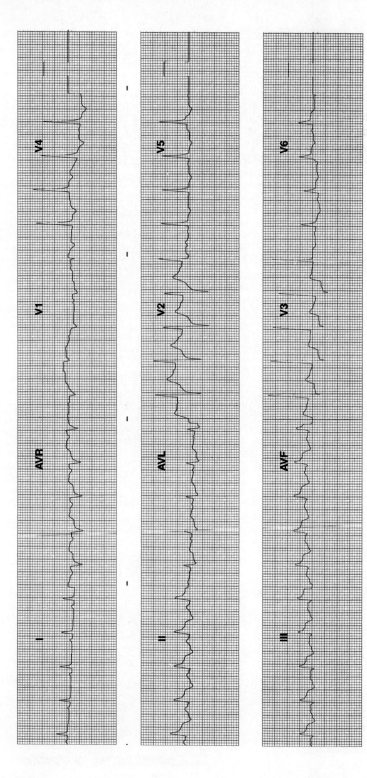

The PR interval is normal. The QRS interval appears wide and might be read as left bundle branch block. If the QRS is carefully inspected, it is noted that the QRS interval is normal. The elevated ST segments and significant Q waves in the inferior leads represent an acute inferior infarction. The ST depression in the anterior leads represents the reciprocal changes of infarction and may masquerade as widened QRS complexes. Sinus tachycardia is present at 114 per minute. The QRS axis is +60°. No other abnormalities are present.

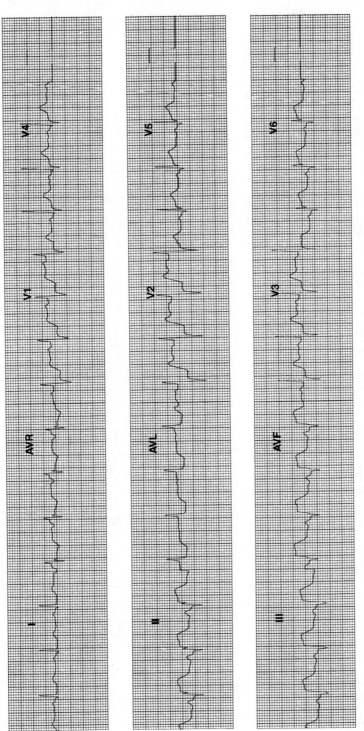

The PR and QRS intervals are normal. The QRS interval appears to be widened in many of the leads. This is caused by the ST elevation of infarction and the ST depression representing the reciprocal changes of infarction. There is sinus rhythm at 88 per minute. The QRS axis is 0°. Left atrial enlargement and right atrial enlargement are absent. Left ventricular hypertrophy and right ventricular hypertrophy are not evident. No hemiblocks are present. There are significant Q waves both in the inferior and lateral leads. Both infarctions are diagnosed as acute because of the elevated ST segments accompanying them.

DIFFERENTIAL DIAGNOSIS

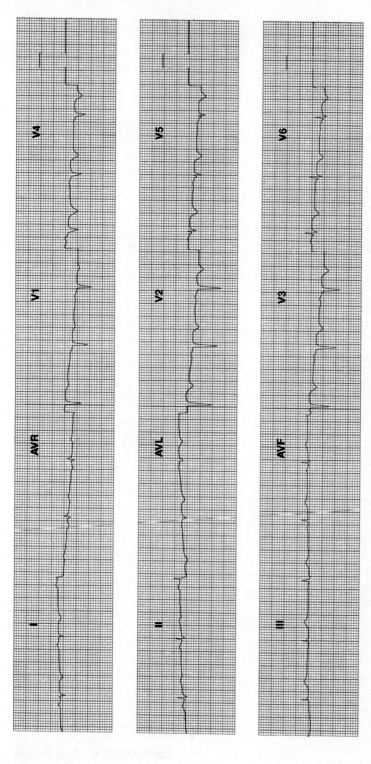

The PR and QRS intervals are normal. There is sinus rhythm at 66 per minute. The QRS axis is +120°. Left atrial enlargement and right atrial enlargement are absent. Left ventricular hypertrophy and right ventricular hypertrophy are not present. The right axis of +120° suggests the diagnosis of left posterior hemiblock, but the axis is rightward because of the anterolateral infarction. The age of the infarction is indeterminate because of the inverted T waves.

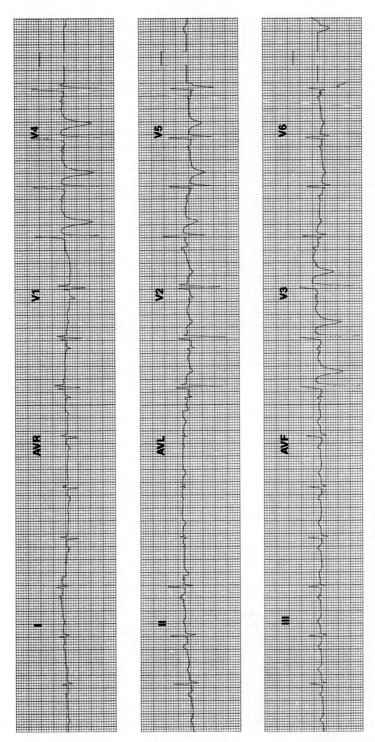

The PR and QRS intervals are normal. There is sinus rhythm at 78 per minute. The axis is +60°. Left atrial enlargement is present. Neither left ventricular hypertrophy nor right ventricular hypertrophy is indicated. Hemiblocks are absent. No significant Q waves are present, but deeply inverted T waves in the anterolateral leads indicate ischemia. These T waves are deeply inverted enough to diagnose ischemia rather than nondiagnostic ST-T abnormalities.

DIFFERENTIAL DIAGNOSIS

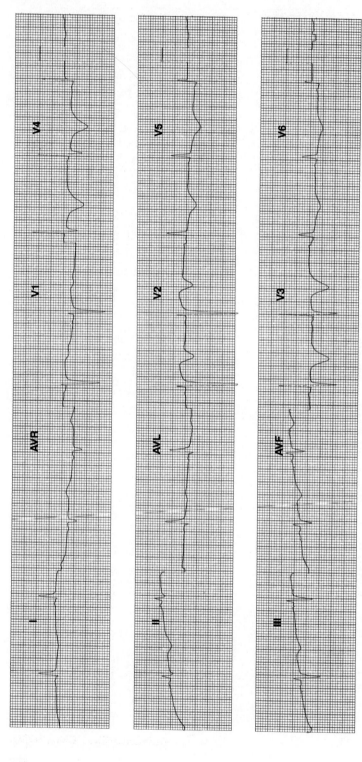

The PR and QRS intervals are normal. Sinus bradycardia is present at 52 per minute. The QRS axis is −15°. Left atrial enlargement and right atrial enlargement are absent. Neither left ventricular hypertrophy nor right ventricular hypertrophy is diagnosed. No hemiblocks are present. No significant Q waves are seen, but throughout the tracing, there is ST depression and deep T wave inversion consistent with ischemia.

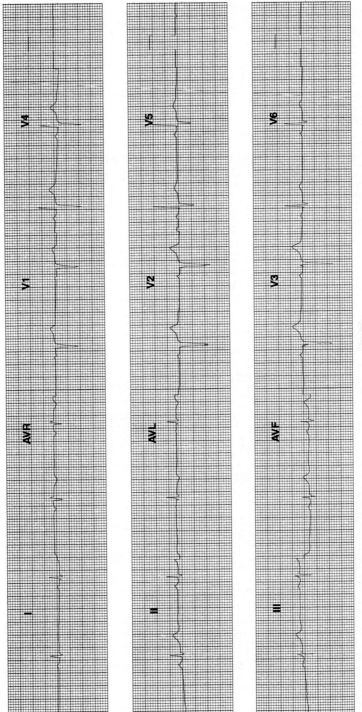

The PR and QRS intervals are normal. There is sinus bradycardia at 49 per minute. The QRS axis is +30°. No enlargements or hypertrophies are seen. Hemiblocks are absent. An old anterior infarction is present with significant Q waves in leads V_1–V_3. Lateral T wave abnormalities are seen, but are not conclusive enough to be diagnosed as ischemic.

DIFFERENTIAL DIAGNOSIS

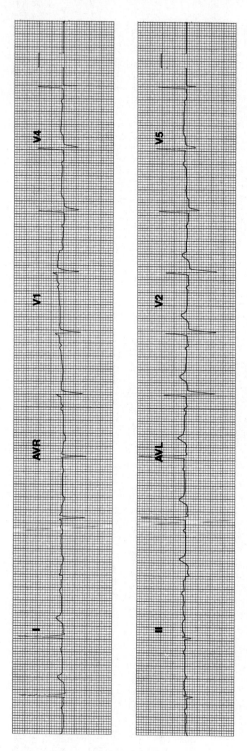

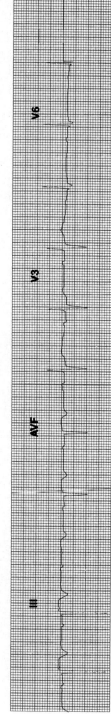

First degree AV block is present. The QRS interval is normal. Sinus rhythm is present at 64 per minute. The QRS axis is −40°. No enlargements or hypertrophies are present. The axis is left because of significant Q waves in the inferior leads, ruling out left anterior hemiblock. An inferior infarction is diagnosed and because the ST segments are elevated in the inferior leads accompanied by T wave inversion, an acute infarct is diagnosed. The ST-T changes present in the anterior and lateral leads are not significant enough to be diagnosed as ischemia.

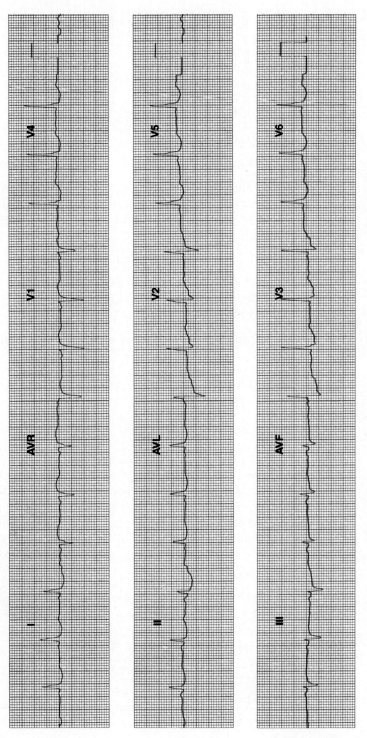

The PR and QRS intervals are normal. There is sinus rhythm at 79 per minute. The QRS axis is 0°. No enlargements or hypertrophies are present. Hemiblocks are absent. Significant Q waves are not present. Nondiagnostic anterolateral ST-T abnormalities are present.

DIFFERENTIAL DIAGNOSIS

Miscellaneous Effects. Electrolyte disturbances and drug effects are only suggested on an ECG and the ability to diagnose these miscellaneous effects is often contingent on serial ECGs and clinical correlation. But we will try to suggest certain abnormalities or at least offer differential diagnoses.

The flattened T wave and the presence of a U wave lead one to suspect hypokalemia. But often the U wave is superimposed on the T wave, and the effect is that of quinidine with a marked QT prolongation and ST-T abnormalities.

The slim-peaked or tent-shaped T waves of hyperkalemia, best seen in the precordial leads, are more easily diagnosed. But patients with posterior wall infarctions and even normal individuals may show a similar pattern.

Hypocalcemia is best diagnosed by a prolonged ST segment and is often seen in conjunction with hyperkalemia. Although the QT interval is prolonged, as in quinidine effect, the ST segment is clearly the cause of the lengthening.

Hypercalcemia is diagnosed by a shortened QT interval, caused by a shortened or absent ST segment.

Digitalis effects are characterized by downward sloping or scooping of the ST segment and a flattened or inverted T wave. These changes are easily confused with repolarization changes of hypertrophy or ischemic changes.

Pericarditis and early repolarization have the same diagnostic criteria on an ECG, but one is considered a normal variant and the other is indicative of disease. The ST segment elevation of pericarditis displays a concave curvature, and the elevation is usually throughout the tracing. In early repolarization the ST elevation is noted especially in the left precordial leads. The ability to obtain previous and serial ECGs, along with clinical correlation, is the best indicator of pericarditis.

The ST segment elevation of an acute infarction can also simulate pericarditis. If the ST elevation is noted in leads with significant Q waves, it is assumed that they represent the ST segment elevation of an acute infarct.

Reversed arm leads on an ECG tracing can resemble dextrocardia in the limb leads, but the precordial pattern will remain normal. True dextrocardia has both the limb leads and precordial leads taking on a characteristic pattern.

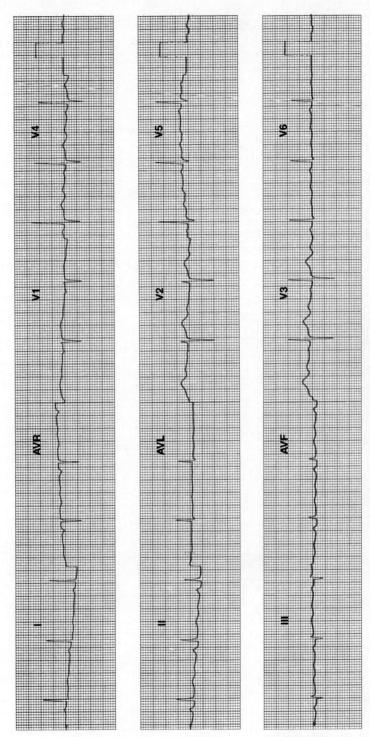

The PR and QRS intervals are normal. There is sinus rhythm at 65 per minute. The QRS axis is 0°. No enlargements or hypertrophies are present. Hemiblocks are absent. There are no significant Q waves. A definite U wave can be seen in most leads, and with the flattened T wave a diagnosis of hypokalemia is suggested.

DIFFERENTIAL DIAGNOSIS

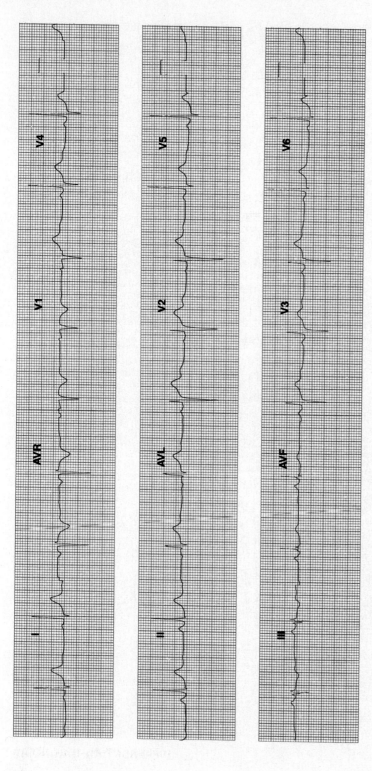

The PR and QRS intervals are normal. There is sinus bradycardia at 54 per minute. The QRS axis is +30°. No enlargements or hypertrophies are present. Hemiblocks are absent. No significant Q waves are seen. A U wave can be recognized in most leads, leading to the suggestion of hypokalemia.

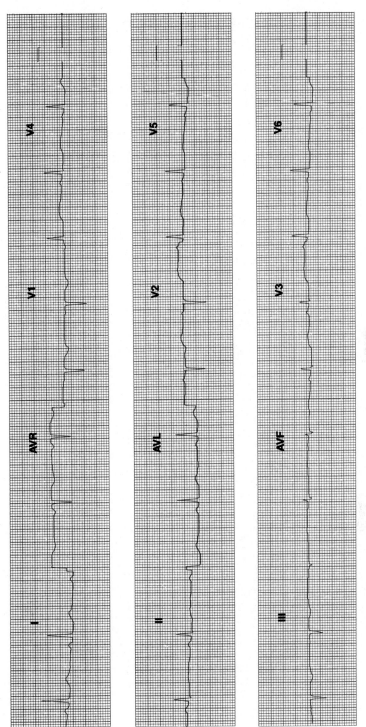

The PR and QRS intervals are normal. There is sinus bradycardia at 58 per minute. The QRS axis is 0°. No enlargements or hypertrophies are seen. Hemiblocks are absent. Poor R wave progression in leads V_1 and V_2 suggests an anteroseptal infarction, age indeterminate. A long QT interval is noted with nonspecific ST-T abnormalities, suggesting quinidine effect.

DIFFERENTIAL DIAGNOSIS

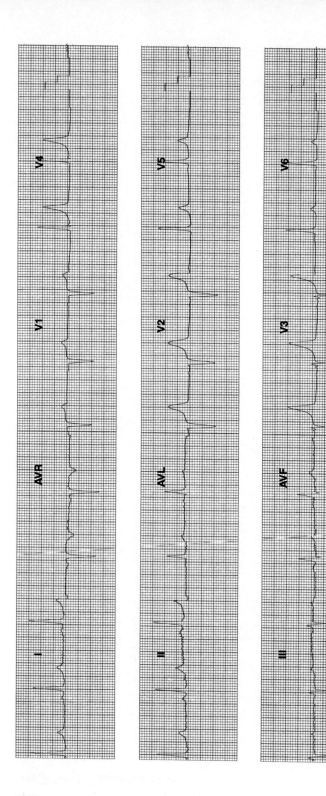

The PR and QRS intervals are normal. Sinus bradycardia is present at 58 per minute. The QRS axis is +30°. Left atrial enlargement and right atrial enlargement are absent. Left ventricular hypertrophy is present. No hemiblocks are diagnosed. A probable old anteroseptal infarction is present because of the poor R wave progression. The T waves are peaked throughout the entire tracing, suggesting hyperkalemia.

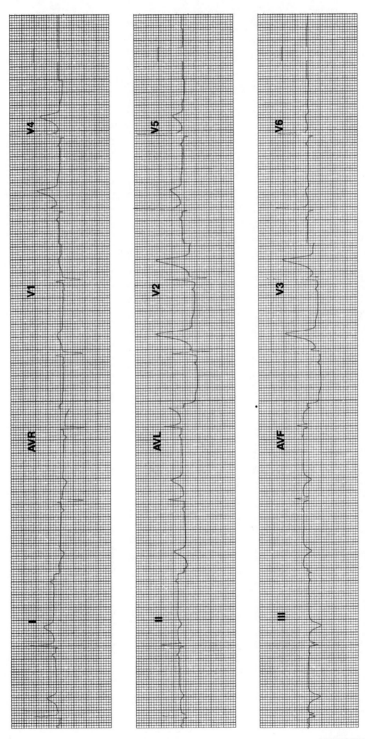

The PR and QRS intervals are normal. There is sinus bradycardia at 53 per minute. The QRS axis is 0°. No enlargements or hypertrophies are seen. No hemiblocks are present. An inferior infarction, age indeterminate is diagnosed by the significant Q waves noted and the inverted T waves. There is a tall R wave in lead V$_2$ accompanied by a tall T wave, indicating a probable posterior wall infarction. The tall peaked T waves are not those of hyperkalemia because they only occur in leads V$_2$ and V$_3$ but are probably attributed to the posterior infarction.

DIFFERENTIAL DIAGNOSIS

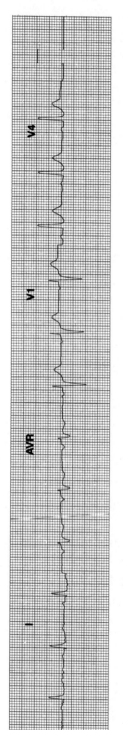

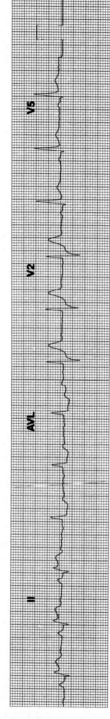

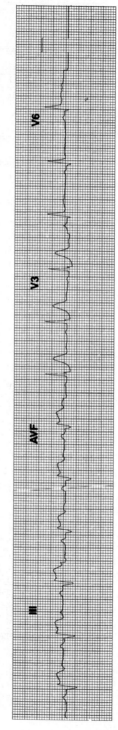

The PR and QRS intervals are normal. There is sinus rhythm at 73 per minute. The QRS axis is 0°. No enlargements or hypertrophies are present. No hemiblocks are diagnosed. The significant Q waves and ST elevations in leads II, III, and aVF allow us to diagnose an acute inferior infarction. Leads V_1 and V_2 contain tall R waves, ST depression, and tall T waves, confirming the diagnosis of a posterior infarction. The tall T waves are attributed to the posterior infarction and not hyperkalemia.

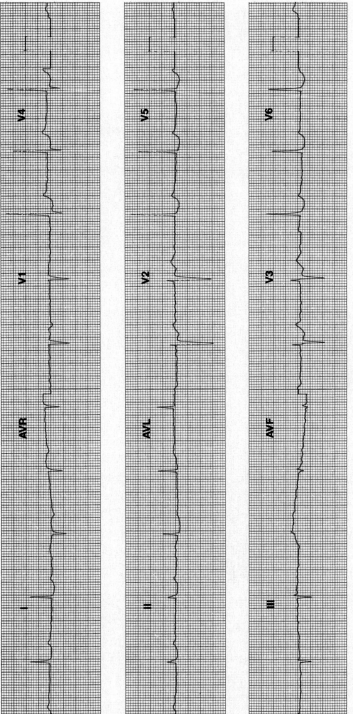

A probable junctional rhythm is present at 60 per minute. The QRS interval is normal. The QRS axis is 0°. No enlargements or hypertrophies are diagnosed. Hemiblocks are absent. An old inferior infarction is probable. The ST scooping in leads with tall R waves is highly suggestive of digitalis effect.

DIFFERENTIAL DIAGNOSIS

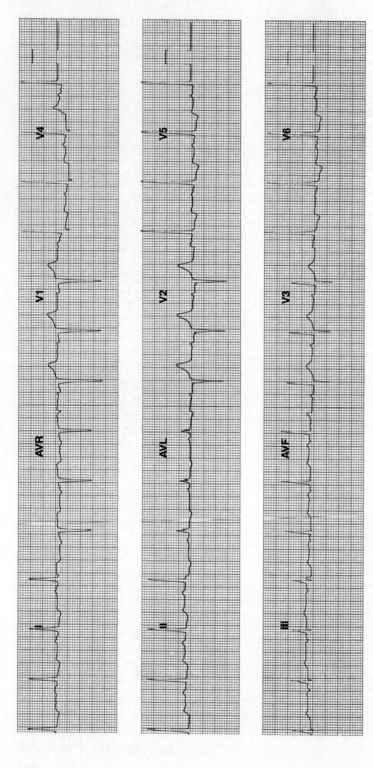

The PR and QRS intervals are normal. There is sinus rhythm at 78 per minute. The QRS axis is +60°. Left atrial enlargement is present. Left ventricular hypertrophy is present. An old anteroseptal infarction is diagnosed. The ST-T abnormalities, as best seen in the leads with tall R waves, represent the repolarization changes of left ventricular hypertrophy. No ST scooping of digitalis is seen.

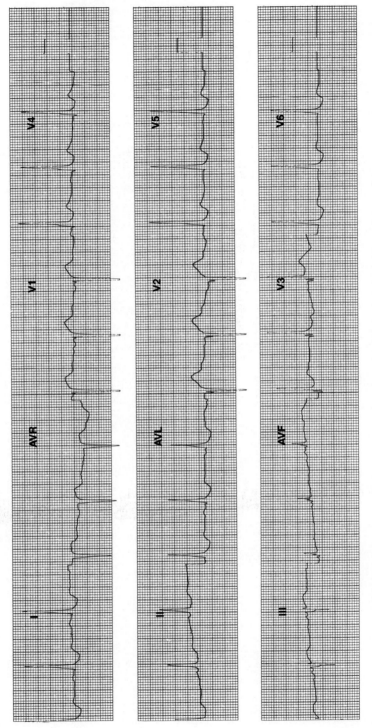

The PR and QRS intervals are normal. There is sinus rhythm at 70 per minute. The QRS axis is 0°. Neither left atrial enlargement nor right atrial enlargement is present. Left ventricular hypertrophy is diagnosed. Significant Q waves are absent. Although there are repolarization changes of left ventricular hypertrophy, there is diffuse ST segment sagging, suggesting digitalis effect.

DIFFERENTIAL DIAGNOSIS

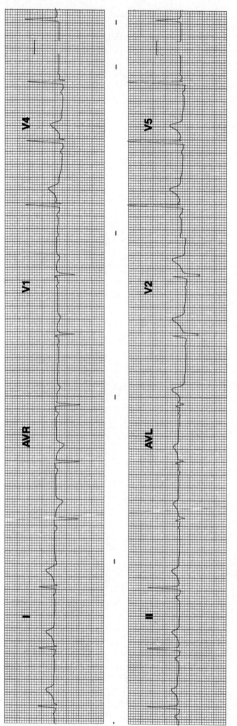
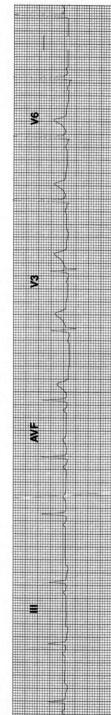

The PR and QRS intervals are normal. There is sinus rhythm at 62 per minute. The QRS axis is +60°. No enlargements or hypertrophies are present. Hemiblocks are absent. No significant Q waves are present. There is ST elevation in the precordial leads, and the patient is a man, aged 22, indicating that this is probably early repolarization rather than pericarditis.

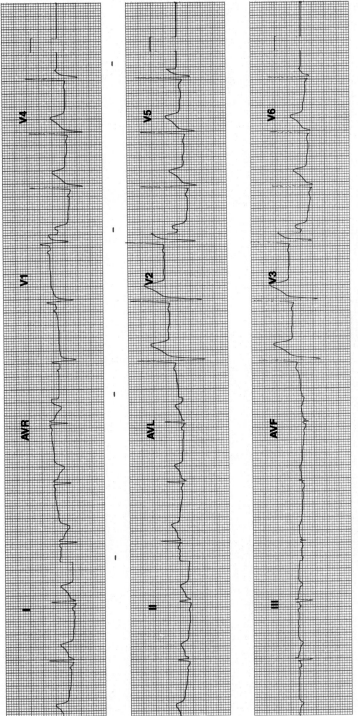

The PR and QRS intervals are normal. There is sinus rhythm at 66 per minute. The QRS axis is 0°. No enlargements or hypertrophies are present. Hemiblocks are absent. No significant Q waves are seen. There is widespread ST elevation demonstrating probable pericarditis.

DIFFERENTIAL DIAGNOSIS

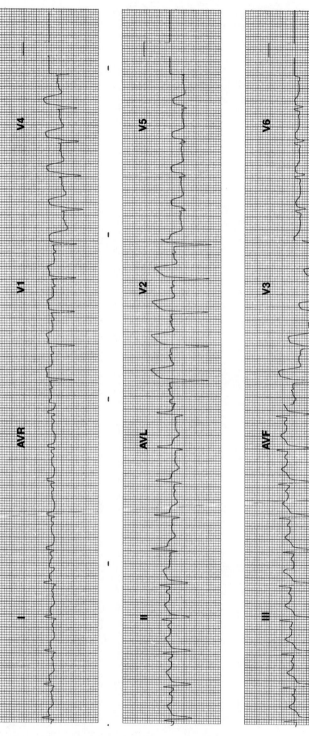

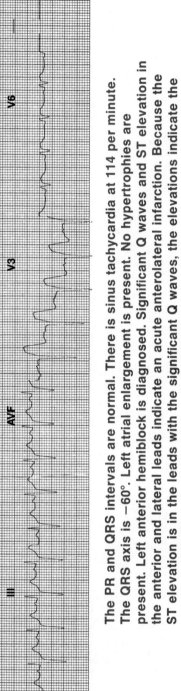

The PR and QRS intervals are normal. There is sinus tachycardia at 114 per minute. The QRS axis is −60°. Left atrial enlargement is present. No hypertrophies are present. Left anterior hemiblock is diagnosed. Significant Q waves and ST elevation in the anterior and lateral leads indicate an acute anterolateral infarction. Because the ST elevation is in the leads with the significant Q waves, the elevations indicate the acuteness of the infarction and do not represent pericarditis.

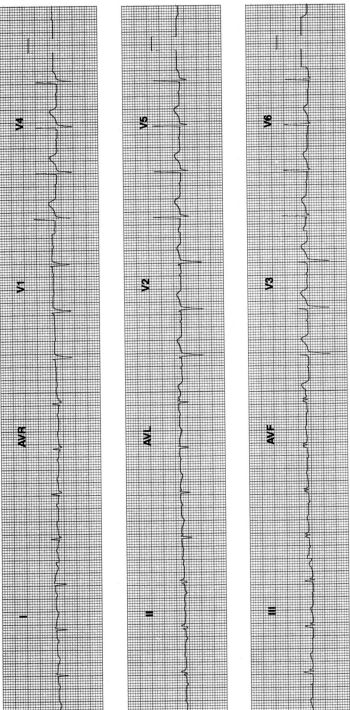

The PR and QRS intervals are normal. You should be immediately aware that both the P wave and QRS complex are negative in lead I and upright in lead aVR. This suggests reversed arm leads or dextrocardia. To meet the criteria for dextrocardia, the R waves in the precordial leads would become increasingly smaller in leads V_1–V_6 as the leads move away from the heart on the right side of the chest cavity. In this tracing, the R wave progression is normal, making it evident that the limb leads are reversed, and dextrocardia is not present.

DIFFERENTIAL DIAGNOSIS

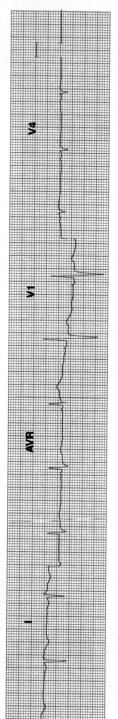

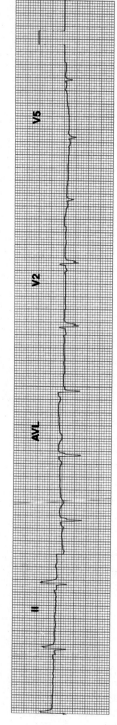

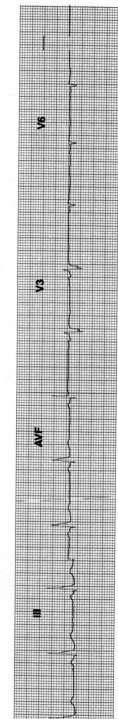

The PR and QRS intervals are normal. You should be immediately aware that both the P wave and QRS complex are negative in lead I and upright in lead aVR. This suggests reversed arm leads or dextrocardia. If this were a case of limb lead reversal, the precordial lead configurations would be normal. This ECG demonstrates dextrocardia. The R waves in the chest leads become progressively smaller as they move away from the heart, which is positioned abnormally in the right side of the chest cavity.

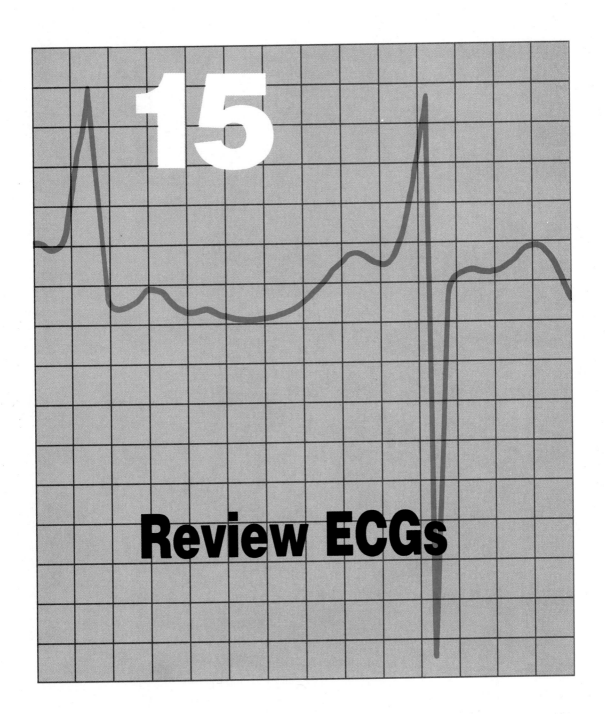

15

Review ECGs

On the following pages is a collection of 25 ECGs illustrating the ECG abnormalities discussed in the preceding chapters. The review ECGs will enable you to practice your interpretation skills and to determine correct differential diagnoses. The answers will be found at the end of the chapter.

REVIEW ECG 1

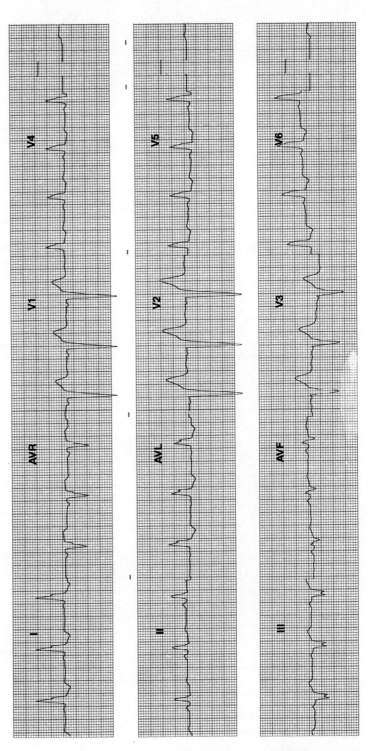

REVIEW ECG 2

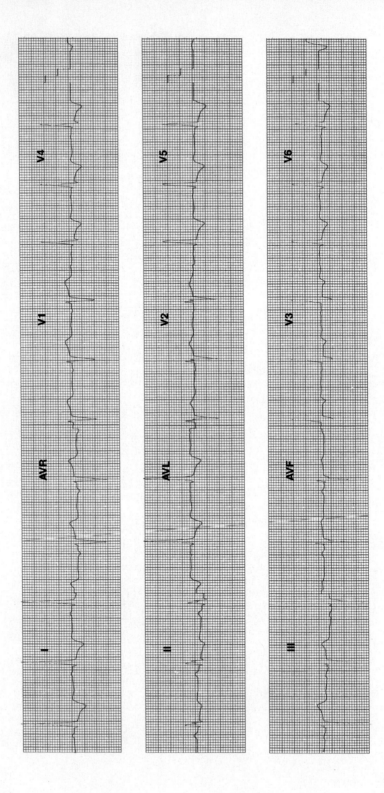

REVIEW ECG 3

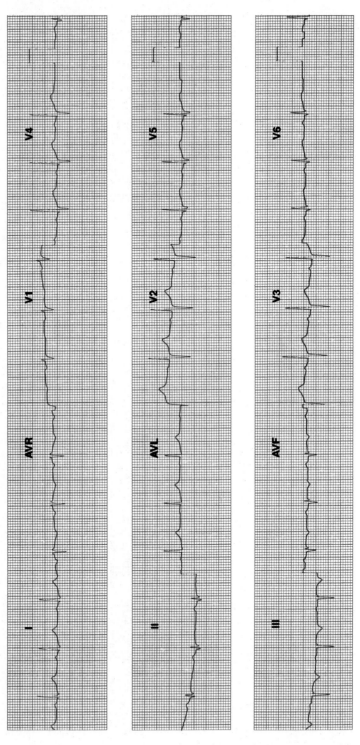

REVIEW ECG 4

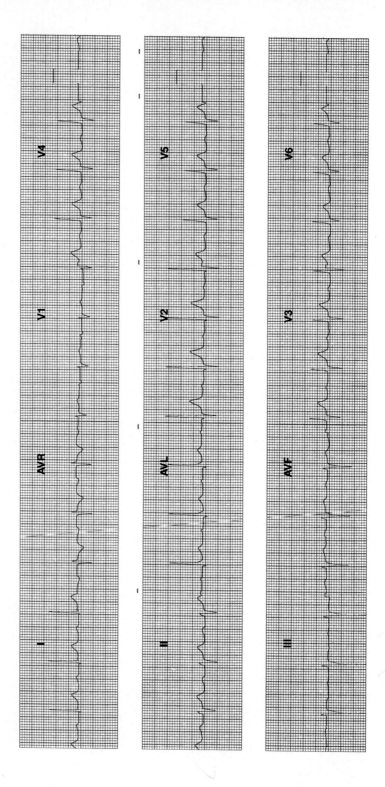

REVIEW ECG 5

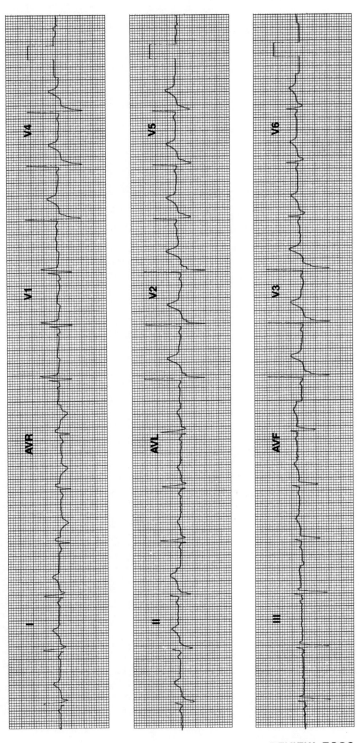

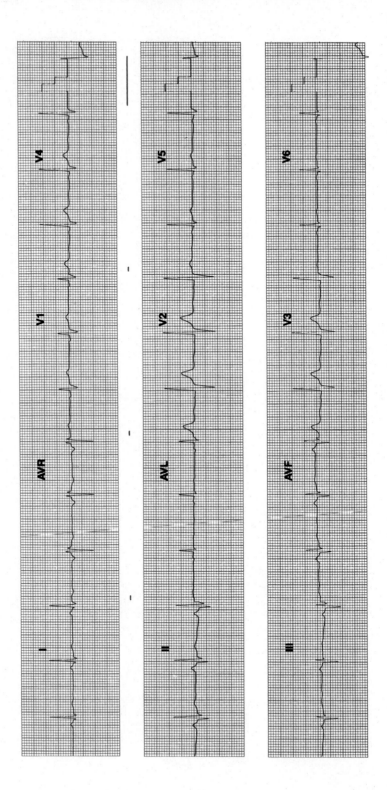

REVIEW ECG 7

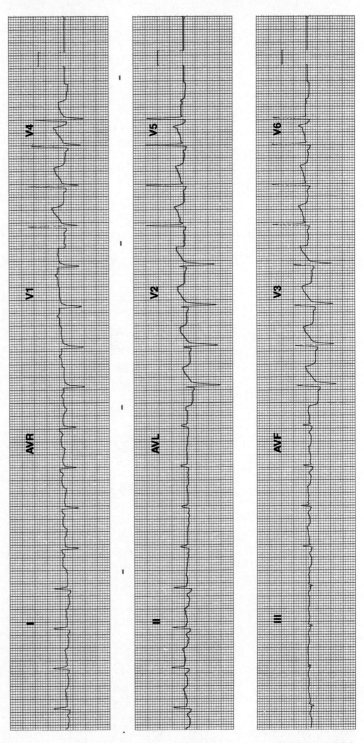

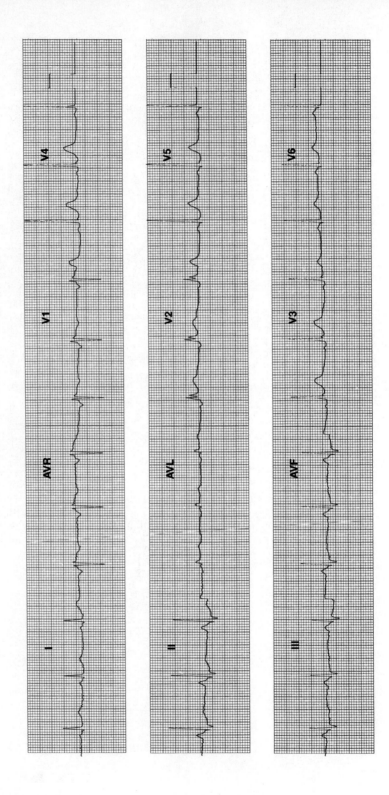

REVIEW ECG 9

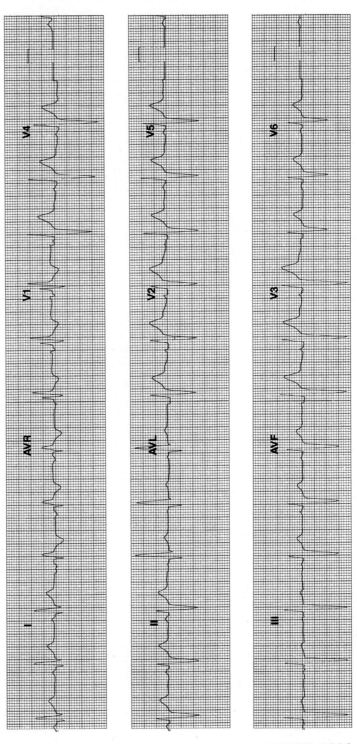

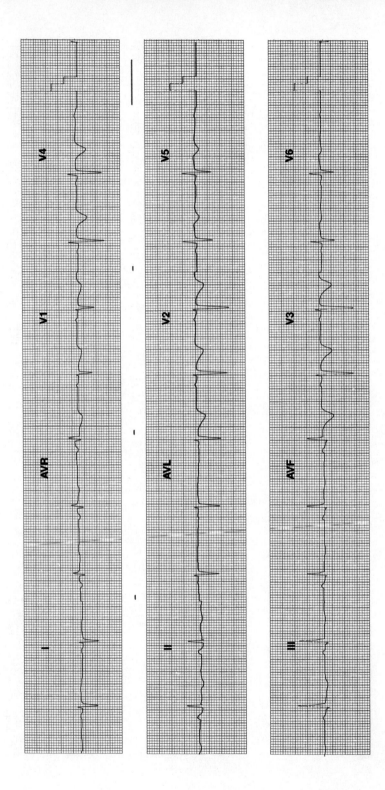

REVIEW ECG 11

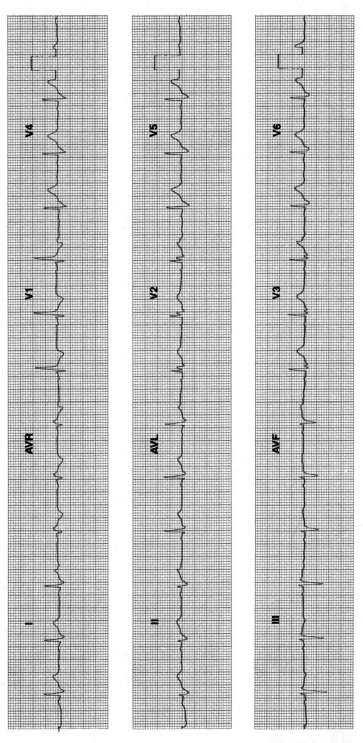

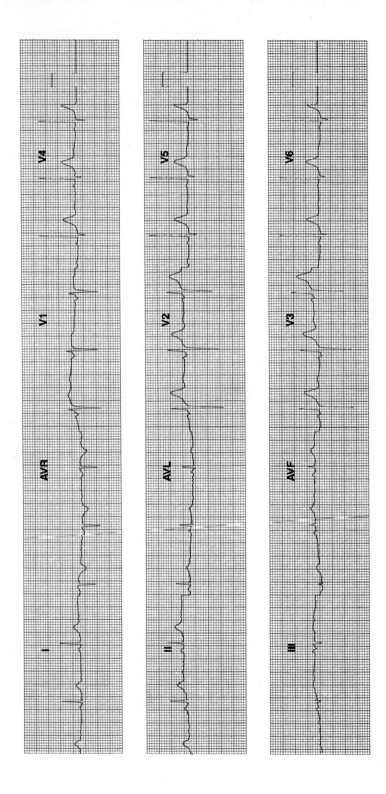

REVIEW ECG 13

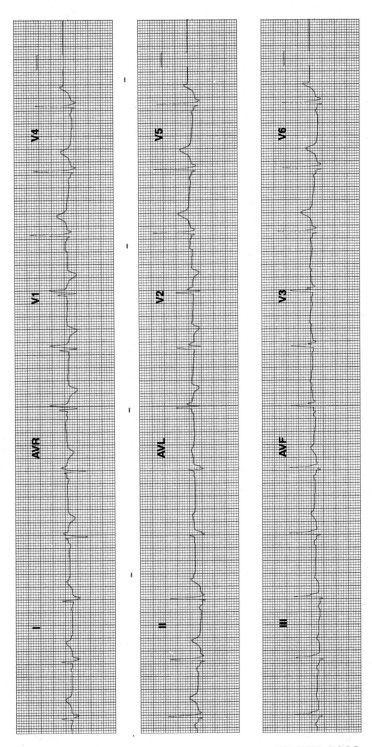

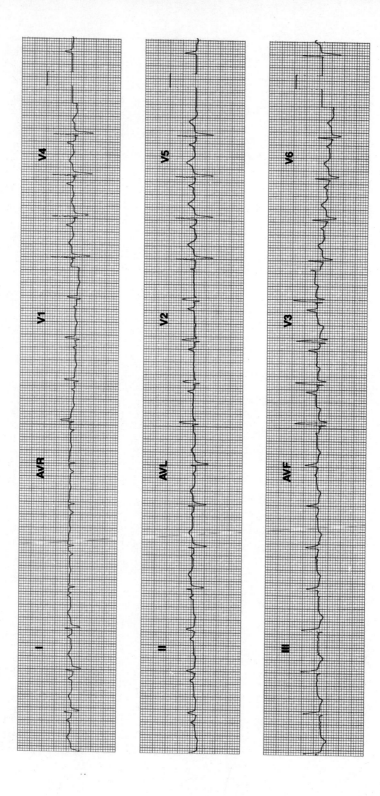

REVIEW ECG 15

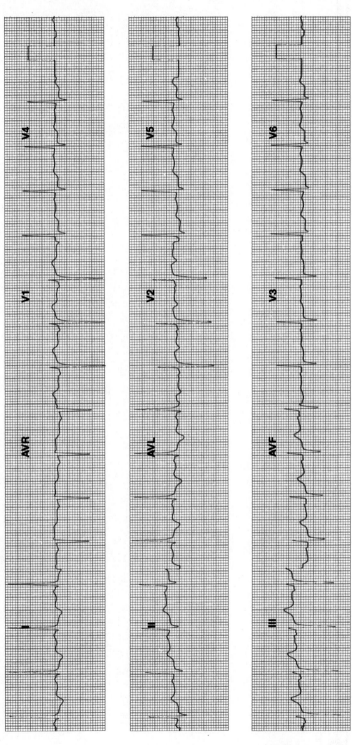

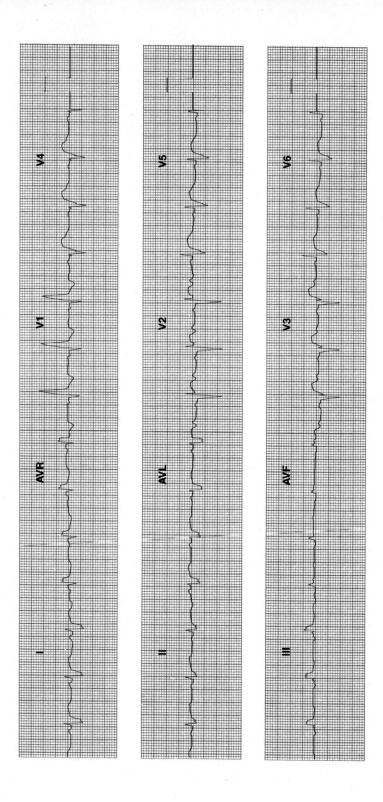

REVIEW ECG 17

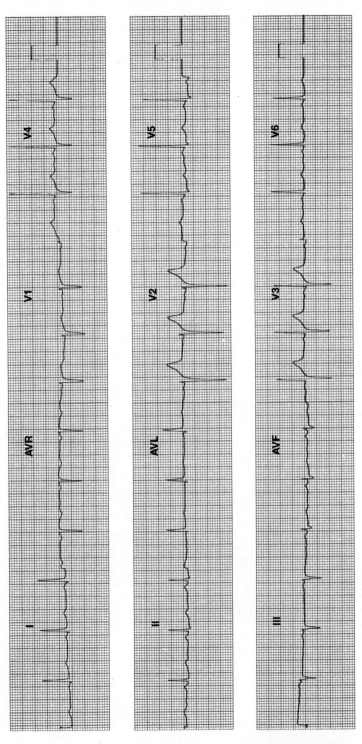

REVIEW ECG 18

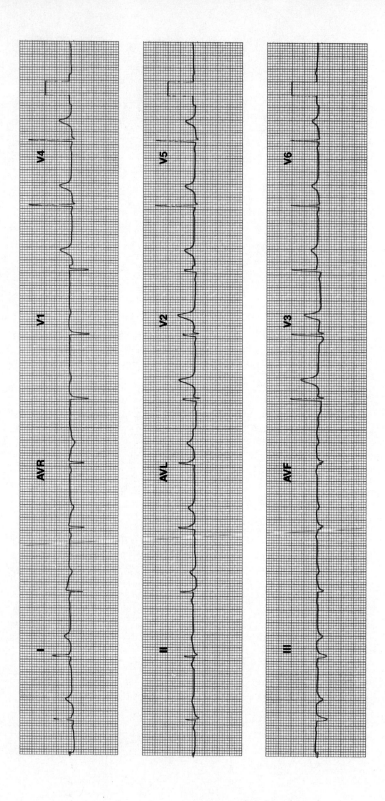

REVIEW ECG 19

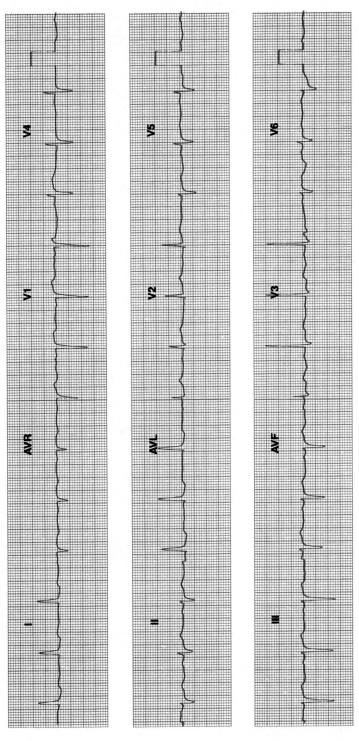

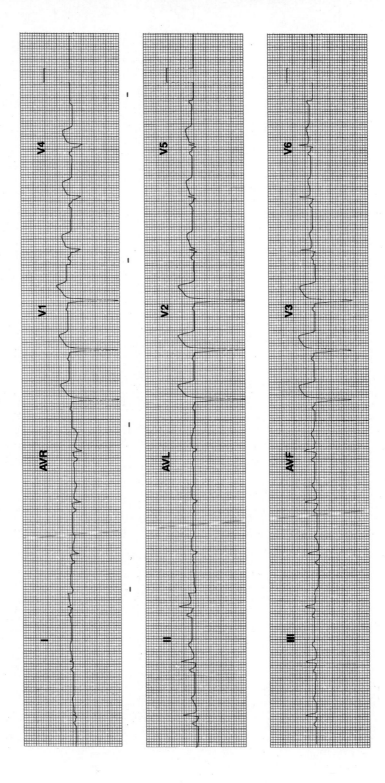

REVIEW ECG 21

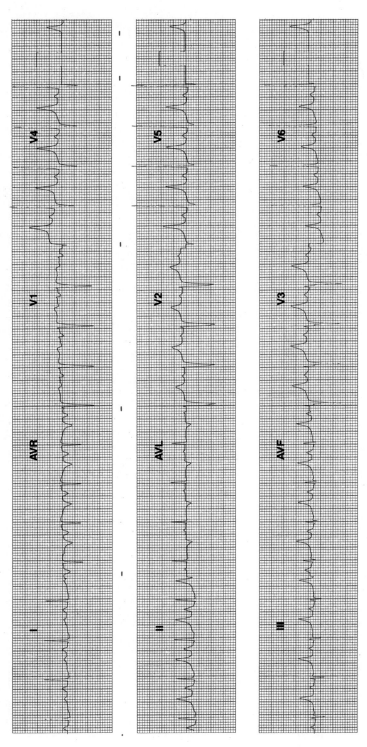

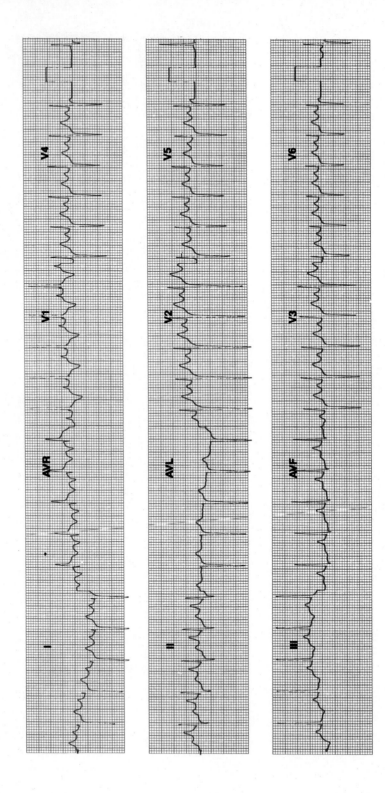

REVIEW ECG 23

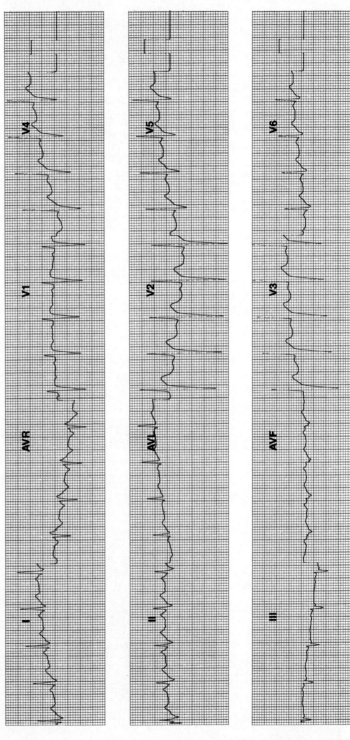

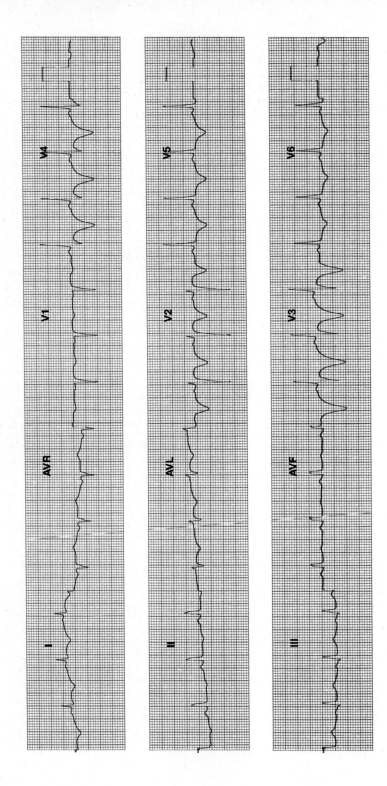

REVIEW ECG 25

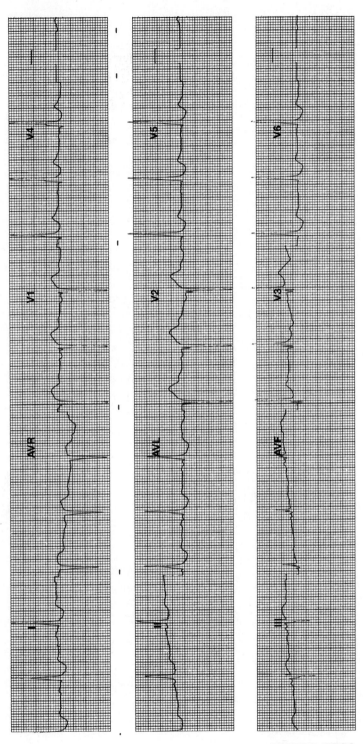

REVIEW ECG ANSWERS

1. Sinus rhythm with left bundle branch block
2. Sinus rhythm with left ventricular hypertrophy
3. Sinus rhythm with an inferior infarction, age indeterminate
4. Sinus rhythm with first degree AV block and left anterior hemiblock
5. Sinus rhythm with right bundle branch block and left anterior hemiblock
6. Sinus rhythm with an old inferior and posterior infarction
7. Sinus rhythm with diffuse ST elevation—probable pericarditis; one atrial premature contraction noted
8. Sinus rhythm with biatrial enlargement and nondiagnostic ST-T abnormalities
9. Sinus rhythm with left atrial enlargement, left ventricular hypertrophy, right bundle branch block, left anterior hemiblock, and an old lateral infarction
10. Sinus bradycardia with left posterior hemiblock and anterolateral ischemia
11. Sinus rhythm with right bundle branch block and left anterior hemiblock
12. Sinus rhythm with left atrial enlargement
13. Sinus rhythm with right bundle branch block
14. Sinus rhythm with right ventricular hypertrophy
15. Sinus rhythm with left ventricular hypertrophy
16. Sinus rhythm with right bundle branch block, left posterior hemiblock, and an acute anterior infarction
17. Sinus rhythm with nondiagnostic ST depression
18. Sinus rhythm with an inferior and posterior infarction, age indeterminate
19. Sinus rhythm with left anterior hemiblock and nondiagnostic lateral T changes
20. Sinus rhythm with acute anterior and lateral infarctions
21. Sinus rhythm with biatrial enlargement and probable hyperkalemia and hypocalcemia
22. Sinus tachycardia with right atrial enlargement and right ventricular hypertrophy
23. Sinus tachycardia with a nonspecific intraventricular conduction disturbance
24. Sinus rhythm with anterior and lateral ischemia
25. Sinus rhythm with left atrial enlargement, left ventricular hypertrophy and possible digitalis effect

BIBLIOGRAPHY

Chung E: Electrocardiography, 2d ed. Philadelphia, Harper & Row, 1980

Dubin D: Rapid Interpretation of EKG's, 3d ed. Tampa, Cover Publishing, 1978

Goldman MJ: Principles of Clinical Electrocardiography, 11th ed. Los Altos, Lange, 1982

Mangiola S, Ritota M: Cardiac Arrhythmias. Philadelphia, JB Lippincott, 1974

Marriott H: Practical Electrocardiography, 7th ed. Baltimore, Williams & Wilkins, 1983

Netter F: Ciba Collection of Medical Illustrations, Vol 5, The Heart. Rochester, Case–Hoyt, 1981

Rosenbaum M, Elizari M, Lazzari J: The Hemiblocks. Oldsmar, Florida, Tampa Tracings, 1970

INDEX

INDEX

left, 121–122, 126
right, 127

T wave (*continued*)
in ischemia, 193–194, 328
in left ventricular hypertrophy, 293
in left ventricular repolarization, 123
in myocardial infarction, 327
inversion of, 200, 201, 202
posterior, 222–223
normal configuration of, 66
in pediatric ECG, 252–253
in twelve-lead ECG interpretation, 95–111
in ventricular repolarization, 26
Twelve-lead ECG
interpretation of
accurate tracing and, 90–92
artifacts and, 93–94
guide for, 95
standardization and, 94–95
Twelve-lead system
Einthoven's triangle in, 4, 90
electrode placement in, 3
lead configuration, 58–59
limb leads in
augmented, 5–6, 59, 63–64
standard, 3–4, 58, 63–64
precordial leads in, 6–7, 63, 64
vectors in
of atrial depolarization, 56–57
mean, 56–58, 65
of ventricular depolarization, 60–62

Unipolar lead(s). *See* Augmented limb leads; Precordial leads
U wave
in hypokalemia, 236–237, 254–255
in ventricular repolarization, 26

Vector(s)
of atrial polarization, 56–57
mean
atrial, 56–58
ventricular, 65
of ventricular depolarization, 60–62, 65, 121, 122
mean, 65
Velocity, of conduction, 11
Ventricle(s)
left, 14, 16, 17
right, 14, 16
Ventricular activation time, 27–28
Ventricular depolarization. *See under* Depolarization
Ventricular hypertrophy. *See under* Hypertrophy
Ventricular repolarization. *See under* Repolarization
Voltage(s)
measurement of, 32–33
in QRS complex, 71–73, 79
standardization of, 94–95
in ventricular hypertrophy
left, 123
right, 127

Wave(s). *See also specific wave, e.g. P wave*
deflection of, 28–29
in depolarization
atrial, 57–58
ventricular, 63–64
duration of, 34
positive and negative, 28–29